The Innocent Eye

PHILOSOPHY OF MIND

SERIES EDITOR: David J. Chalmers, Australian National University and New York University

Self Expression
Owen Flanagan

Deconstructing the Mind
Stephen Stich

The Conscious Mind
David J. Chalmers

Minds and Bodies
Colin McGinn

What's Within?
Fiona Cowie

The Human Animal
Eric T. Olson

Dreaming Souls
Owen Flanagan

Consciousness and Cognition
Michael Thau

Thinking Without Words
José Luis Bermúdez

Identifying the Mind
U.T. Place (author), George Graham, Elizabeth R. Valentine (editors)

Purple Haze
Joseph Levine

Three Faces of Desire
Timothy Schroeder

A Place for Consciousness
Gregg Rosenberg

Ignorance and Imagination
Daniel Stoljar

Simulating Minds
Alvin I. Goldman

Gut Reactions
Jesse J. Prinz

Phenomenal Concepts and Phenomenal Knowledge
Edited by Torin Alter, Sven Walter

Beyond Reduction
Steven Horst

What Are We?
Eric T. Olson

Supersizing the Mind
Andy Clark

Perception, Hallucination, and Illusion
William Fish

Cognitive Systems and the Extended Mind
Robert D. Rupert

The Character of Consciousness
David J. Chalmers

Perceiving the World
Edited by Bence Nanay

The Contents of Visual Experience
Susanna Siegel

The Senses
Fiona Macpherson (editor)

Attention is Cognitive Unison
Christopher Mole

Consciousness and the Prospects of Physicalism
Derk Pereboom

Introspection and Consciousness
Edited by Declan Smithies and Daniel Stoljar

The Conscious Brain
Jesse J. Prinz

Decomposing the Will
Edited by Andy Clark, Julian Kiverstein, and Tillmann Vierkant

Phenomenal Intentionality
Edited by Uriah Kriegel

The Peripheral Mind
István Aranyosi

Does Perception Have Content?
Edited by Berit Brogaard

The Innocent Eye
Nico Orlandi

The Innocent Eye

Why Vision Is Not a Cognitive Process

NICO ORLANDI

OXFORD
UNIVERSITY PRESS

OXFORD
UNIVERSITY PRESS

Oxford University Press is a department of the University of Oxford. It furthers the University's objective of excellence in research, scholarship, and education by publishing worldwide.

Oxford New York

Auckland Cape Town Dar es Salaam Hong Kong Karachi Kuala Lumpur Madrid Melbourne Mexico City Nairobi New Delhi Shanghai Taipei Toronto

With offices in

Argentina Austria Brazil Chile Czech Republic France Greece Guatemala Hungary Italy Japan Poland Portugal Singapore South Korea Switzerland Thailand Turkey Ukraine Vietnam

Oxford is a registered trade mark of Oxford University Press in the UK and in certain other countries.

Published in the United States of America by
Oxford University Press
198 Madison Avenue, New York, New York 10016

Library of Congress Cataloging-in-Publication Data
Orlandi, Nico.
The innocent eye : why vision is not a cognitive process / Nico Orlandi.
pages cm
ISBN 978-0-19-937503-5 (hardback)
1. Vision–Philosophy. 2. Visual perception. I. Title.
B105.V54O75 2014
152.14–dc23 2013044596

1 3 5 7 9 8 6 4 2
Printed in United States of America
on acid-free paper

A Fiorella, Donato e Lele

Contents

Acknowledgments

I NEVER THOUGHT I was going to write a book. Then things got out of hand. I found myself writing longer and longer papers without quite saying what I wanted to say about vision. Before I realized it, I slipped into book mode. I do not know if I managed to say it all in *The Innocent Eye*, but I hope I managed to say it somewhat better.

I do not think that this book contains many novel ideas. I tried to verbalize (ideally in a clear way) what some others in philosophy and the cognitive sciences have been thinking about perception in recent years and in the history of these disciplines. Some of the central notions of the book—for example some of the distinctions that concern the notion of representation—started to become clear when I was a graduate student in the Department of Philosophy at UNC-Chapel Hill. I cannot properly express how grateful I am to have been able to study there. I thank my mentors, Bill Lycan and Jesse Prinz, as well as my unofficial mentors, Dorit Bar-On, Ram Neta, Jay Rosenberg, Mike Resnik, and Geoff Sayre-McCord, for teaching me so much about philosophy and beyond. While at UNC, I also benefited enormously from conversation with a number of fellow graduate students. This work would not have seen the light without their insight, and I can safely call them my teachers: Matthew Chrisman, Elizabeth Foreman, Nancy Lawrence, Felipe de Brigard, Bryce Huebner, Eric Mandelbaum, Ted Parent, Mark Bauer, David Landy, Dylan Sabo, Susanne Sreedhar, and others. Thanks to Dylan Sabo for illuminating analysis of both concept-acquisition and mental representation. Thanks to Eric Mandelbaum for inferences, associations, and the Fodorian point of view.

My colleagues at Rice University provided invaluable help and constructive criticism. Among them, I need to mention and thank Charles Siewert for being an example of how philosophy should be done, George Sher for all of his wisdom, and Casey O'Callaghan for so much good philosophy, friendship, loyalty, and everything else. Thanks also to a past member of the Rice department, Eric Margolis, for encouragement and advice. Thanks to David Velleman for being an excellent mentor and a fantastic friend. An advanced version of the manuscript was read by Todd Ganson as well as in a seminar in philosophy of perception that I co-taught with Casey O'Callaghan at Rice in the fall of 2013. Thanks to Todd and to the seminar participants for helpful comments.

Although I did not particularly love the criticism at the time, I am also grateful for the work of a number of anonymous referees at both Oxford University Press and MIT Press. Their reports were incredibly helpful. I believe they made the book much better. One of the referees who chose to identify herself, Susanna Siegel, deserves special mention for her support, for detailed comments, and for being an all-around role model. The acquisition editors of both Presses, Peter Ohlin, Lucy Randall, and Philip Laughlin, as well as the production editor at Oxford University Press, Marc Schneider, have been exemplars of professionalism and efficiency. I thank them for their hard work.

The Innocent Eye could not have been written without the help of the Stanford Humanities Center and the Rice Humanities Research Center. I thank, in particular, Katja Zelljadt and Robert Barrick of the Stanford Humanities Center for making it pretty much impossible not to work. Thanks to Jessica Williams and Graciela De Pierris of the Stanford Department of Philosophy for useful comments on some of the material of chapter 4. I also own gratitude to Springer Science and Business Media, John Wiley and Sons, and Taylor & Francis for kind permission to reproduce passages from previous articles. Parts of this book were published in *Nous, Phenomenology and the Cognitive Sciences, Philosophical Psychology*, and *Review of Philosophy and Psychology*.

I am forever grateful to the parentheses-hater Jenny Judge for taking care of the figures, for editing advice, and for excellent comments. Thanks to Austin Jarvis for figure 3.2. Thanks to Natalie for teaching me Latex and many more good things in life. Finally, I thank all of my friends and family for making it all worthwhile.

List of Figures

1

Vision is not a cognitive process

The sort of mentation required for perception is (. . .) not different in *kind*—though no doubt it differs a lot in conscious accessibility—from what goes on in Sherlock Holmes' head when he infers the identity of the criminal from a stray cigar band and a hair or two. If what Holmes does deserves to be called cognition, perception deserves to be called cognition too, or so, at least, some psychologists like to say.

(FODOR 1984, p. 31)

1.1 Introduction

Why does the world look to us as it does? When we look around we typically see a rich panorama of objects and their properties. We see items that have specific shapes, colors, and sizes and we generally see them as preserving these properties through changes in illumination and distance from the observer. But why do we see the world this way rather than some other way? Why do objects appear to preserve their dimensions despite changes in the size of their retinal projection? Shouldn't we see them shrink as their projection also shrinks? These questions are at the heart of the study of vision.[1] They ask for an explanation of how vision produces the perceptions that we commonly enjoy rather than some other ones.

In vision science, a number of answers have been offered to these questions that vary significantly in detail. Despite the variation, we can divide the answers into two general camps that have been particularly active in the last fifty or so years.[2] This distinction may have fuzzy boundaries, and it may be difficult to judge, in individual cases, which camp a particular theory belongs to. What is relevant is that these are two fairly recognizable camps, and the position developed in this book falls pretty clearly on one side of this divide.

1. Koffka 1935.

2. For this way of dividing the camps, see Palmer 1999, p. 47.

According to the first camp, the world looks the way it does because we *construct* it to look as it does. Perceivers make an essential contribution, in particular a *cognitive* contribution, to how the world appears. Visual percepts, in this framework, are the product of an unconscious *inference* or an unconscious *interpretation*.[3] This view has been proposed, among others, by David Marr and Irvin Rock and, although I later argue that this is problematic, it is seemingly also accepted by proponents of Bayesian accounts of perception. It is a view that centers mostly on the subject or the individual, and it is regarded as a form of intellectualism where implicit 'knowledge' is used to interpret visual inputs.[4]

According to the second camp, by contrast, the world looks to us the way it does primarily because of how the world *is*. Analyzing the environmental conditions under which vision occurs together with organismic facts about our brains and visual *apparati* is sufficient to explain how we perceive. The observer's cognitive contribution is not necessary. This camp has its roots in the work of J. J. Gibson and, although it can still be considered a minority camp in cognitive psychology, some of its fundamental ideas have garnered support among philosophers of perception.[5]

The contrast just drawn between subject-centered and world-centered approaches is of course in need of further spelling out. Neither party to the debate denies that the way the world is plays a role in explaining how we perceive it to be. Neither party denies that our visual apparatus, typically understood as comprising retina, optic nerve, and visual cortex, makes an essential contribution to seeing. Nevertheless, the two camps disagree on the need to appeal to further explanatory resources. Subject-centered views suppose that making reference solely to environmental conditions and to physiological and functional facts about perceivers is insufficient. Visual perception consists of an unconscious reconstruction of the scene where visual percepts are derived in steps, and in a regimented fashion, from other *representational* material. In particular, ignoring differences of detail, inferential accounts presume that vision makes use of both more basic *sensory representations* and some encoded

---

3. 'Inference,' 'construction,' and 'interpretation' are used interchangeably by proponents of cognitive accounts, and I explain below in greater detail what these different terms mean. Unless otherwise noted, I also use the terms interchangeably. See Clark 2012, Gregory, 1970, Howhy et al. 2008, Maloney and Mamassian 2009, Mamassian et al. 2002, Marr 1982, Palmer 1999, Rescorla forthcoming, Rock 1983, von Helmholtz 1924.

4. Noë 2004.

5. Chemero 2009, Gibson 1966, 1979, Hurley 2002, Noë 2004, Rowlands 1999.

assumptions to deliver stable percepts. The assumptions constitute the implicit 'knowledge' of environmental contingencies that is distinctive of inferential accounts. World-centered views, by contrast, deny that it is necessary to think of vision this way.

In this book, I favor a version of this second, world-centered view. I argue that vision is not a cognitive activity and that the visual system is not a cognitive system because, in many paradigmatic cases, we do not need to appeal to representations to explain what vision does. I argue for this position with an argument to the best explanation. We can explain the central phenomena that we need to explain by thinking of the visual process as mediated by functional states and features that are better understood non-representationally, and by making reference to environmental conditions, in particular to statistical regularities in the world with an eye to organismic needs. This approach, I claim, is more compatible with current research on vision, and it is overall more plausible on both empirical and theoretical grounds.

I start, in the next chapter, by sketching a picture of visual processing where the intermediate steps of the process are understood in non-representational terms. This picture requires, first, the idea of a system that is biased or naturally constrained or wired to perform certain operations.[6] These different terms mean that a system may have features—for example, wires or constraints—that developed, and continue to develop, under evolutionary and environmental pressure. These features have a certain function. They make the system act lawfully; that is, they make the system act in a way that is describable by principles. The principles, however, are in no sense represented by the system and encoded within it. To think of the features as representational elements amounts to ascribing representations too liberally.

To make clear that the internal features are not representational elements, I speak of visual systems as 'relying on environmental facts.' Relying on a fact means acting in accordance with a fact, and with a corresponding principle, without representing either. The fact itself enters into an explanation of what the system does without being encoded by the system. In my terminology, wired (or biased or constrained) systems are systems that rely on environmental facts. To highlight the role that the environment plays for such systems, I also call them 'embedded' or 'situated' systems, and I call the resulting view

6. This idea is already present in the work of a number of cognitive scientists and philosophers. I propose to take it seriously, and to take seriously the idea that encoded assumptions in vision are not assumptions at all. For this idea, see Burge 2010, p. 404, Dennett 1991, Piccinini 2008a, Pylyshyn 1984, 1999, p. 354, Ramsey 1997, See also Orlandi 2011b and the work of Dylan Sabo on concept acquisition in, for example, Sabo unpublished and 2013.

the embedded view (EV). Connectionist and neural networks will later serve as useful examples of embedded systems.

The next step in my argument is to show that early and intermediary sensory states are also not representations. There is, in general, some disagreement concerning the function of such states.[7] One of the insights of recent Bayesian accounts of perception is that early vision is not (or not primarily) in the business of informing about proximal conditions—for instance, conditions of the light affecting the retina.[8] The primary function of early vision is to signal error or the discrepancy between what is expected and what is given. This may suggest that sensory states, although perhaps representing error, do not perform a representational function as traditionally understood. They do not inform concerning a condition external to the system in which they operate.

But even if we subscribe to a classical way of understanding sensory states—that is, even if we view them as detectors—I think that we should resist thinking of them in representational terms. This is because we need to draw a distinction between representations and functional states that are merely sensitive to the environment. Intermediate visual states are tracking states.[9] They are primarily active within a restricted domain (visual processing) and they merely respond reliably to what they causally and statistically correlate with. They are not sufficiently *de-coupled* from their causal origin, where de-coupleability is one of the conditions for representational status.

The remainder of the book is dedicated to showing that this picture is empirically and theoretically plausible. I argue that the distinction between sensitivity and representational capacity is both needed and already supported by a good portion of philosophy and cognitive science (chapter 3). I then move on to demonstrate the explanatory power of the embedded view by offering models of multistability, completion, misperception and other central visual phenomena (chapter 4). I conclude with a chapter on the notion of computation (chapter 5). The embedded view I favor, and ecological views

7. See Akins 1996 for an example of skepticism regarding the idea that sensory states play a detector function.

8. See section 2.4.

9. The idea of a tracking state is also present in the work of a number of theorists who reflect on the notion of representation, and I suggest in section 3.3 that it is accepted also by theorists who allegedly hold very minimal accounts of representation. For the idea of a tracking or responding state (the terminology varies) see Burge 2010, Cantwell-Smith 1996, Clark and Toribio 1994, Cummins and Poirier 2004, Dretske 1997, Fodor 1987b, Pylyshyn 1984, Ramsey 2007, See also the work of Sabo on concept acquisition. Sabo unpublished and 2013.

more generally, are compatible with computationalism. The development of new kinds of computational systems is precisely what inspires non-cognitive understandings of the visual act. Such development makes room for a new outlook on vision that is often overlooked and that we have no reason to dismiss.

Overall, I think that the field of vision science has moved toward an ecological approach of the kind I defend. Models of vision in Natural Scene Statistics, discussed in chapter 2, as well as work in connectionism and neural networks, and reflection on the notion of representation support an embedded approach to vision. For this reason, I find it puzzling that a good portion of the field retains the old terminology. Bayesian views, in particular, are typically classified as inferential and I treat them as such in the present chapter. I ultimately argue, however, that they are compatible with an embedded outlook.

Preserving the old terminology is often the result of holding overly liberal accounts of mental representation. I argue that deflated notions are misguided and that they trivialize what it means for a state or feature to represent the environment. Such notions perpetuate misunderstandings by giving the impression of keeping an inferential account of perception, while the real sense of inference is, in fact, lost.

Defending a world-centered view means favoring an anti-intellectualist understanding of the visual act. Seeing objects that preserve their properties through change does not require an inference: it does not presuppose knowledge, implicit or explicit, of environmental contingencies. The eye is able to form percepts by simply responding adaptively to the environment that we inhabit. The eye is, in other words, innocent.[10]

Although the claim that we do not need inferences and representations to explain visual activity is recognizably Gibsonian, the position defended here is also different from classical ecological accounts in at least two respects. First, the position I defend is an intermediary position because I hold that, even though vision is not itself a cognitive *process*, its *products* are plausibly cognitive. I hope to make clear that once we reflect on the notion of mental representation, we can suppose that, while later stages of visual processing are representations, the process that generates them does not itself make use

10. The eye is also biased in various ways, but when I talk of the eye's innocence I am referring to the fact that, if the embedded view is right, then seeing does not presuppose a construction that deploys cognitive resources. Seeing is innocent because it is not dependent on an inference, but it is biased and constrained in various other ways by environmental contingencies and by the role of attention. See section 4.8.

of representational states. Vision is a direct, yet representational, response to the environment.

Further, in providing an embedded understanding of vision I do not appeal to the notion of *action* and to the role of movement in perception (more on this in section 1.4). Action and perception obviously interact in various interesting ways. I aim to show, however, that, even if we work under the idealization that vision is a static process, we should accept an embedded, rather than a cognitive understanding of it.

In this introductory chapter, I clarify the main thesis and argument of this book. Since my main thesis is that vision is not a cognitive process, section 1.2 starts by explaining what a cognitive process is and offers a preliminary characterization of what mental representations are. The section also provides some context by giving examples of theories of perception that are constructive in the sense of presuming that vision is mediated by representations. Section 1.3 sketches the argument of the book, while section 1.4 looks at some of the consequences of accepting the world-centered account proposed here and places the current project within recent literature in philosophy and the cognitive sciences.

1.2 The thesis

This book proposes the view that vision is not a cognitive activity and that the visual system is not a cognitive system. Since these claims may strike many as odd we should start by clarifying what this thesis means.

In the subsections that follow, I suggest that a plausible way to think of cognitive systems and processes is to suppose that they trade in mental representations. I also give a preliminary characterization of what representations are, classifying different historical accounts as more or less *committal*. I then show that some contemporary theories of vision are cognitive in the relevant sense, focusing in particular on the fairly common claim that vision is inferential. The main thesis of the book then emerges as the view that while visual perception *produces* representational states, it does not *use* representations in doing so.

Cognitive systems and mental representations

The word 'cognitive' is used in various different ways in the psychological sciences. Occasionally, it is used to mean 'non-perceptual' or 'theoretical' and it is used to draw a contrast between perceptual mental operations and non-perceptual ones.[11] Other times, the term is used to describe areas of the brain that control non-perceptual functions—for example, pre-frontal cortex. It is also not uncommon to use it as a synonym for 'mental.'[12]

Nevertheless, there is a central sense of the term whereby a cognitive system or process is understood to trade in mental representations. Cognitive systems differ from other kinds of systems—for example, from mechanical or biological or functional systems—not just in their complexity but also because they require explanatory notions that are proper to psychology. Cognitive systems traffic in mental representations.[13]

This claim can amount to a thesis that is more or less robust: one may think that a system is cognitive because it *issues* mental representations, or that it is cognitive because it also *uses* mental representations. Both of these ideas are present in vision science and to better understand them we need to first grasp what mental representations are.

Representation: first look (committal and deflationary notions)

Although the notion of representation has been often at the center of dispute, I think that the description that I propose here captures the basic distinctive features of mental representations and can be found in the theories of otherwise disagreeing philosophers and cognitive scientists of both the past and of the present. Mental representations are basic explanatory posits of psychology. Like other explanatory notions of the empirical sciences, they are unobservable entities and their presence and characteristics can only be inferred through the behavior that they supposedly bring about and explain.

Representations are *mental* insofar as they are distinctive of psychology. They are, in this sense, different from *conventional* representations such as maps, paintings, photographs, signs, and stories, although they may share a number of features with them. As theoretical posits, representations[14] are typically introduced to explain the behavior and capacities of a system when appeal to environmental and other conditions fails, or is not illuminating.[15]

11. Pylyshyn 1999.

12. Clark and Grush 1999.

13. Fodor 1984, Fodor and Pylyshyn 1988, Pylyshyn 1984, Ullman 1979, p. 6.

14. Unless otherwise noted, the term 'representation' refers in this book to mental representations rather than to conventional ones.

15. Brooks 1991, Burge 2010, Fodor 1987a, 1987b, Fodor and Pylyshyn 1988, James [1890]1983, Pylyshyn 1984, ch. 2, Segal 1989, Van Gelder 1995.

Zenon Pylyshyn makes this position explicit when he writes:

> (. . .) it should again be emphasized that the notion of representation is necessary only in the context of explanation; it is needed to state generalizations concerning the behavior of systems under certain descriptions.(. . .) Thus, if under a particular description of a system's behavior, a physical, neural, or purely functional account capture all the relevant generalizations hence serves the explanatory function, then appealing to representations is not essential.
>
> (Pylyshyn 1984, p. 26)

Appeal to representations is justified if it helps explain behavior, and, as Pylyshyn remarks, this is typically the case when behavior is considered *under a particular description*. Behavior can be described in various ways. It can be described, for example, in terms of the specific *movements* that a system, agent, or organism performs. Alternatively, behavior can be described in terms that ignore details of implementation. Walking to the door can be done in various specific ways, with different specific movements that are not captured by the general description 'walking to the door.'

While a *complete* physics would presumably be able to account for *all* generalizations that concern movement, representations figure in explanations that concern behavior described at a fairly abstract level, a level that ignores details of how the behavior is carried out.[16] Representing someone to be at the door figures in an explanation of walking to the door that does not mention either how the walking specifically takes place or how the representation is implemented in the brain. Representations, like behaviors, are *multiply realizable* and they are defined, at least in part, *functionally*, or by how they affect performance.

Similarly, when it comes to subsystems of a whole person or organism, *their* behavior (or performance) can be described at various levels of abstraction.[17] If we follow David Marr, we can give a description at the 'task level' that specifies what a system—for example, the visual system—does, in general terms. At this level, we abstract from both details of implementation and

---

16. Dennett 1987, ch. 2 Fodor 1987a. A *complete* physics should be able to predict the output of any organism, and of anything in the universe, described in physical terms. The idea is that non-physical notions, such as the notion of representation, are required when events are described at a different level of abstraction.

17. Marr 1982, ch. 1.

from procedural details—that is, from how a system goes about performing its task at both the algorithmic and the hardware levels. In the case of vision, we want to know how the visual system produces stable percepts with stable properties despite variations in the light hitting the eye. This explanation requires both the specification of a procedure for how this task is carried out and a specification of the neuronal structures that carry it out in the brain. Cognitivism about perception and the embedded competitor I present in this book are theories of the procedure that vision carries out.

Representations are derivatively fairly abstract functional notions that help explain behavior under a certain description. Representations are also a specific subset of functional notions. As it will be apparent later in the book, not all functional states and features of a system are representations. Representations are introduced when appeal to *environmental* conditions is not illuminating and they have some distinctive features that allow them to perform this characteristic function. Described at a fairly general level, the features are:

1. Standing in,[18]
2. Informing, and
3. Guiding performance.

Representational structures *stand in* for something other than themselves and in so doing they act as *mediators* within a system or a process. Additionally, representations are special kinds of mediators: they are *semantic* mediators. They *inform* about an entity, property, or state of affairs typically (but not exclusively) external to the system in which they occur. What it means for something to inform is a matter of dispute. Accounts of information vary from purely causal accounts to probabilistic accounts. What is further required for a state to inform *selectively* is also a matter of dispute (more on this in section 3.3). Despite these disagreements, however, the general consensus is

---

18. I borrow the terminology of standing *in* from Clark 1997, p. 144 and Haugeland 1998, ch. 8. This terminology has intentional connotations, but I use it here to capture the idea that representations are internal *intermediaries* that we appeal to in the context of explaining behavior. I typically speak of what the representation is about in terms of what it stands *for* or what it stands *in for*. 'Standing in' and 'standing in for', as I intend them here, are different from their homonyms in Grush 1997. Although I agree with Grush on many aspects of the distinction between presentation and representation, he uses 'standing in' as a mark of something that functions as a simulator—that is, as something that can be used off-line as a model. I do not follow his use here. Standing in is meant to just point to the role of representations as mediators.

that representations are states that inform. Finally, representations are *causally active* semantic mediators, guiding the behavior of a system or organism, described in certain general terms, by standing in and informing.

As *informants*, mental representations say something about what they stand in for and they have *content*. To a first approximation, the content of a representation is given by what the representation represents.

This characterization of content is ambiguous and it reflects a noted ambiguity in the notion of content itself. We can think of contents on the model of the contents of a bucket, or on the model of the contents of a newspaper.[19] Perceptual representations and other mental attitudes, such as beliefs, are typically thought to have content in the latter sense. They are states that convey information in a similar fashion to how a newspaper does—for example, by saying that the world is some way or other, or by saying that something is present here and now.

Because they convey information in this sense, the content of perceptual representations is identified with their accuracy conditions. What the representation says specifies the conditions under which the representation is accurate, and what it says can generally be correct or incorrect. When representations carry incorrect information they are said to misrepresent. As we will see in chapter 3, the capacity to misrepresent is crucial to characterizing perceptual and sensory representations since states that stand for external conditions but that cannot misrepresent are thought to lack genuine content and representational status.[20] Since this book is centered on perception, talk of content often coincides with talk of accuracy conditions, leaving aside the issue of whether some mental states have content in the other sense—that is, on the model of the content of a bucket.

Summarizing: the capacity of representations to *inform* concerning some state of the world is deemed central to their having *content*. Their having content, in turn, is deemed central—particularly in the philosophical literature—to both defining representations and distinguishing them from other kinds of functional states and causal mediators.[21]

In addition to *standing in* and *informing*, representations typically figure in the performance of some seemingly unexplainable task, a task that—under a

19. Siegel 2010.

20. It is a further question whether misrepresentation is, more generally, a condition on representation. Representation of mathematical truths may constitute a counterexample. When we represent mathematical truths what we represent cannot be false. But I do not discuss mathematical cases in what follows. Thanks to Susanna Siegel for raising this point.

21. See Burge 2010, ch. 8.

certain description—seems to require precisely that the performing agent has states that have the features of representations just outlined. We think of a system as representing when its observable behavior seems to result from the manipulation of an internal model of the situation, rather than from the situation itself. The internal model is about something and it informs (correctly or incorrectly) concerning what it is about.

So far, I have talked of performance and behavior in ambivalent terms. Performance and behavior can be described in different ways, but they can also refer to what a whole agent—human or non-human—does, or to what a subsystem of a whole agent does. The visual system, in a sense, performs and behaves in a certain way when it produces stable percepts. The system, however, is only a subsystem of a person. When we talk of representations as performance-guiding states, we might refer to their role in a subpersonal transformation, or to their role in producing person-level behavior (or to both).

Although this is a debated issue to which I return in chapter 3, representations typically occur in a number of contexts—for example, they are stored in memory—and they have some *observable* behavioral effects. This means that, even if they occur in some subpersonal transition, they also tend to inform other systems and to ultimately result in person-level performance. This raises the question of whether states that figure *only* in subpersonal transformations are representations. For the moment, we can sidestep this issue. We should keep in mind that thinking of states that are only active in a subpersonal system as representations requires at least a clear sense that the states in question stand in for something else, and that they have genuine content or accuracy conditions.

Standing in, *content*, and agent-level *performance-contribution* are then some basic features of representations. What more specific attributes internal states and structures need to possess in order to have these features is a matter of dispute, and it depends on how robust a notion of representation one holds. It is useful to distinguish accounts of mental representation by their level of richness. In particular, we can differentiate *committal* from *deflationary* views.

Traditional accounts tend to be *committal*. The Representational Theory of Mind, classically understood, holds that mental representations are states that stand in and inform, but that also have linguistic format. They resemble the words of a language, the Language of Thought.[22] Like words, atomic mental representations can be combined and re-combined to form complex representations. These have combinatorial semantics: what

22. Fodor 1975. While once popular, this committal notion of representation is no longer widespread. We will consider it in relation to perception in chapter 5.

they mean or stand for systematically depends on what their atomic constituents mean or stand for. Complex mental representations of this kind can be like declarative sentences of a language, having propositional format that includes predication and quantifiers.

Still on the committal side, but a bit less robust, is the idea that mental representations resemble conventional maps. Like maps, internal structures can bear some sort of isomorphism to the elements in the environment for which they stand, and, by so doing, the structures enable a system to engage in flexible behavior in the absence of what they stand for.[23] Like city maps that are useful because they stand for something absent, as they reproduce some of the properties and relations of streets and buildings, mental representations are map-like reproductions of environmental and organismic situations. Such representations need not have linguistic form, yet this conception is fairly rich as it requires isomorphism and the reproduction of potentially complex spatial relations.

Deflationary views, by contrast, typically hold that representations are more akin to conventional signs. They resemble the level of mercury in a thermometer that signals the outside temperature. There need be no isomorphism between the mercury and the temperature. What is sufficient is that one state carries information, or has the function of carrying information, about the other where carrying information is spelled out in terms of causal or lawful co-variation.[24] By co-varying lawfully with the outside temperature, the level of mercury carries information about it.

Like their committal counterparts, deflationary views may vary in how rich their account of representation is. At the minimal end of the spectrum, representations may be seen simply as states that carry information about, or lawfully co-vary with, what they stand for. A slightly more committal deflationary view is that representational states have the *function* of carrying information. The level of mercury in a thermometer represents the outside temperature, not just because it lawfully co-varies with it but also because it has the assigned function of doing so.[25]

Deflationary accounts of both kinds are particularly popular in some areas of cognitive neuroscience where neurons that respond selectively to some

23. See Grush 1997, Clark and Grush 1999, Grush 1997, Ramsey 2007, ch. 3. See also Gallistel 1990 and Rescorla 2009a, 2009b for a discussion of different kinds of 'cognitive maps' and of whether such maps resemble linguistic representations.

24. Fodor 1990a, O'Reilly and Munakata 2000, pp. 23–25.

25. Dretske 1991.

environmental quantity are said to detect that quantity and, derivatively, to represent it.[26] Neurons in the human primary visual cortex that are found to be sensitive to the presence of edges are considered edge-detectors or edge-representations.

Regardless of how robust an account one holds, it is plausible to suppose that vision involves representations in the sense that the visual system *produces* them. This position is in line with that of most contemporary vision scientists and it is plausible because, when we see, we seem to be in states that have the basic features of representations. We should look at this idea in a bit more detail.

Visual percepts as representations

Consider the case of a perceiver who sees a red cube. In seeing a red cube a subject is plausibly in a representational state that depicts the world to be a certain way. The state carries information about the cube being red, and the state has content. It can be veridical or 'falsidical,' depending on whether there is a cube, and it is, in fact, red. The subject can find herself in such a state even when the cube is not red, and even in the absence of the cube. If so, the subject misperceives the red cube. Further, the subject's state can be used for tasks such as the guidance of action and the forming of beliefs. One typically forms the belief that a red cube is present based on one's visual perception of the cube. Similarly, one can move to grab a red cube given one's perception of it.[27]

Visual states with the features just outlined are typically called 'visual representations' or 'visual percepts' (or sometimes just 'percepts'). The states are *visual* because they are derived from an accredited receptor system. Representations derived from other systems—for example, from memory—are not visual in this sense. The states are *representations* because they have the other basic attributes of representational states outlined previously.

Thinking of visual states as representations has been questioned both by those who reflect on conscious perceptual experience[28] and by those who reflect on the current best models of perception in the cognitive sciences.[29]

26. Elliffe 1999, Lettvin, Maturana et al. 1959, p. 1951.

27. See also Dretske 2006, pp. 5–7 and Wilson 2010, p. 9 for a similar characterization of what perceiving involves.

28. Brewer 2007, Campbell 2002, Martin 2004, Travis 2004.

29. Chemero 2009, Noë 2012.

Embodied and dynamic theorists recommend that we eliminate the notion of representation from accounts of mental activity. Despite these criticisms, however, the idea that visual percepts are representations remains prominent.

As embodied theorists themselves concede, whether we can do without representations—and whether we can think of percepts in non-representational terms—is an empirical issue. It is generally believed that we have to wait and see how things turn out.[30] We simply don't yet know if we can do without them. Perceptual representations are deemed important in explaining how perception interacts with memory and how it plays a role in higher-order mental processes.

In what follows, I hold as a plausible research hypothesis that visual percepts are representations and focus on the question of what it means to say that they are. At the end of the argument, it will turn out that, once we further reflect on the notion of representation and on the evidentiary standards for ascribing it, the products of vision qualify while the states that precede them do not. Whether, despite this analysis, we should still be skeptical of the conclusion that percepts are representations requires further research and argument. Since representations are explanatory posits, it could be that, in the end, we do not need them to explain the role of perception in other mental competences. I think that this is precisely what we have to wait and see.[31]

Accepting that visual percepts are representational states requires clarifying a number of points. The first point is that percepts do not need to be conscious. In priming, for instance, observers may perceive an item without being aware of having seen anything.

The second point is that perceptual representations need not be objects *to us*. When we see, we represent the world to be a certain way but we do not see the representations themselves. Our access to the world is not mediated in this way. Representational structures simply function within us to explain how we act.[32]

---

30. Chemero 2009, pp. 42–43.

31. With these considerations I do not engage much of the literature on perceptual experience. This is, in part, because I take the subject matter of this book to be somewhat different. I am interested in the ontogenesis of perceptual states that may not be conscious, and may not be *experiences*. I do not take a stance on how experiences (and hallucinations) should be individuated, and I remain neutral on the question of phenomenal content, that is, content that supervenes on phenomenological features of perception. What I aim at establishing is rather that, given some positive idea of what representations are, we have good reason to presume that visual states are representations.

32. Clark and Toribio 1994, p. 413.

Other controversial theses concerning perceptual representations are also not mandatory. We do not need to suppose that perceptual representations are very detailed, or that they come in linguistic or propositional format, or that they are constituted out of concepts. If recent Bayesian models of perception are correct, perceptual representations may be 'probabilistic,' encoding the relative probability of the gist of a scene and filling in the details as needed.[33]

Similarly, visual percepts may be map-like, rather than language-like, not displaying genuine predication and a combinatorial structure.[34] The corresponding perceptual *judgments* may have linguistic format, but the perceptual states themselves need not share that format.[35]

Finally, visual percepts need not have conceptual constituents, where I think of concepts as just special kinds of mental representations. They are representations that are used in a variety of inferential and classificatory tasks.[36] Fairly unsophisticated creatures may have perceptual and representational capacities while lacking concepts.[37]

Having cleared up these points, we can return to the task of clarifying the main thesis of this book. I first suggested that cognitive processes (and systems) are distinctive for trading in mental representations. After giving a preliminary characterization of what representations are, we saw that the claim that vision is cognitive can amount to a thesis that is more or less robust. Vision may be cognitive because it *issues* mental representations, or because it also *uses* mental representations (or because of both of these facts). I then suggested that it is plausible to suppose that vision is cognitive in the first sense. We can suppose that visual percepts are representations. I now turn to the claim that representational states are not only products but also intermediaries of perception.

---

33. Clark 2012, p. 188, Eliasmith 2007. See also Noë 2004, Simons and Rensink 2005, Schellenberg 2010, Simons and Levin 1997, for reasons to be skeptical of the richness of visual content.

34. Rescorla 2009a, 2009b.

35. Accordingly, such states may have accuracy conditions rather than genuine truth-conditions (Austin et al. 1950, p. 112). The difference between accuracy- and truth-conditions can be captured by noticing that linguistic representations are capable of asserting that something is the case and they are truth-evaluable. Maps (and pictures) by contrast do not assert anything and can only be more or less faithful depending on their degree of resemblance or isomorphism to what they represent.

36. Machery 2009, Margolis and Laurence 2007.

37. See Gunther 2003 for a survey of the non-conceptual content debate. See Evans 1982 and Peacocke 1992 for early proponents of non-conceptual content. See McDowell 1996 for a dissenter. See also Dretske 1969 for the idea of *non-epistemic* perceptual states.

P- and s-representational intermediaries: inferences and associations

Just like there are more or less robust accounts of representation, there are also more or less robust cognitive accounts of visual perception. A committal instance of cognitivism is the idea that vision is an inferential (or interpretive, or constructive) process.[38] This view is fairly widespread and there are two versions of it. Each has received some attention in philosophy.

The first is a slightly more dated 'bottom-up' version that finds its precursors in David Marr and Irvin Rock and a more recent proponent in Stephen Palmer. The second is a 'top-down' version that finds its precursors in Helmholtz and Gregory and its present incarnation in Bayesian accounts of perception. As should be apparent shortly, the labels 'bottom-up' and 'top-down' are meant to denote the main direction of the process of inference: in one case, the inference starts from the bottom, while in the other it starts from the top. I begin illustrating this inferential view with a small sample of quotes from its proponents. Stephen Palmer writes:

> The objects that we so effortlessly perceive are not the direct cause of our perceptions. Rather, perceptions are caused by the two-dimensional patterns of light that stimulate our eyes. (...) To provide us with information about the three-dimensional environment, vision must therefore be an interpretative process that somehow transforms complex, moving, two-dimensional patterns of light at the back of the eyes into stable perceptions of three-dimensional objects in three-dimensional space. We must therefore conclude that the objects we perceive are actually interpretations based on the structure of images rather than direct registrations of physical reality.
>
> (Palmer 1999, p. 9)

Along, similar lines, David Marr writes:

> (...) the true heart of visual perception is the inference from the structure of an image about the structure of the real world outside.
>
> (Marr 1982, p. 68)

38. Bechtel 1993, p. 124, Churchland 1989, Fodor 1984, Gregory 1970, Howhy et al. 2008, Marr 1982, Palmer 1999, Rescorla forthcoming, Rock 1983, Ullman 1980. See also Hatfield 2009 (part I) for an informative history of this idea and for some of its challenges.

For the top-down camp, Hohwy et al. write:

> There is growing support of the idea that the brain is an inference machine, or hypothesis tester, which approaches sensory data using principles similar to those that govern the interrogation of scientific data. In this view, perception is a type of unconscious inference. (. . .) This view goes back at least to von Helmholtz (1860) and has been expressed with increasing finess since that time (Gregory, 1998; MacKay, 1956; Neisser, 1967; Rock, 1983). More recently it has been proposed that this intuitive idea can be captured in terms of hierarchical Bayesian inference, using generative models with predictive coding or free-energy minimization.
>
> (Hohwy et al. 2008, p. 2)

Similarly, Richard Gregory writes:

> Perception involves a kind of inference from sensory data to object-reality. Further, behavior is not controlled directly by the data, but by the solutions to the perceptual inferences from the data. This is clear from common experience: if I put a book on a table I do not prod the table first to check that it is solid. I act according to the inferred physical object-table—not according to the brown patch in my eye. So perception involves a kind of problem-solving—a kind of intelligence. Helmholtz spoke of perception in terms of 'unconscious inferences'.
>
> (Gregory 1970, p. 30)

Two questions must be answered about these passages. First, what do these different authors mean when they say that the visual system performs inferences? Second, why do they think that it is necessary to think of vision this way?

With respect to the first question, the initial reaction may be to take these different authors to just speak metaphorically. It is hard to make sense of the claim that visual operations are inferential given their automaticity and their independence from conscious control. Some suppose that inferences are only those transitions from premises to conclusions that are conscious or consciously accessible by an agent. Others presume that for an inference to obtain, a thinker has to take the premises to support the conclusion.[39] Accordingly, we may take the inferential claim to be metaphorical and to simply be that vision can be usefully described as an inference.

---

39. Boghossian 2012, Recanati 2002, Smith and DeCoster 1999, p. 326.

This, however, cannot be quite right. An inferential account of vision is supposed to be a research hypothesis that is distinct from ecological and physiological accounts of the visual act. In order to be such a hypothesis it has to be substantive. However, it is not substantive to say that a system is inferential simply because it can be described as performing inferences. We can usefully describe all sorts of systems as inferential in this sense; rivers, plants, stomachs, and a host of simpler mechanisms, such as thermometers and smoke detectors. We can also be quite successful in predicting their behavior in doing so. Many things act *as if* they perform inferences. In this sense, the visual apparatus would be inferential just because pretty much everything is, which is a fairly uninteresting thesis. We need to understand the claim more robustly, and one way to do so is to suppose that vision is inferential, at a minimum, because it consists in a process that uses mental representations.

As we will see shortly, this proposal accords with what contemporary inferentialists about vision say, and it makes the inferential claim distinctive. Direct and ecological accounts do not deny (or, if they do, they shouldn't) that a fair amount of processing occurs in vision and that this processing can be *described* as an inference. What they typically deny is rather that such processing *is* a genuine inference, in the sense of being a process that consists in a transition between representational states. Vision is direct, according to them, not because it isn't mediated by states of the cerebral cortex, but because it is not mediated by representational states.

The idea then is to understand the claim that vision is inferential in terms of it employing representations. What kind of representations? The first thought is that the visual system employs more basic representations of the stimulus that are easily obtained from the light that reflects on the retina. In seeing a red cube, the visual apparatus uses representations of those elements of the cube that are derivable from its reflectance properties—for example, its rough boundaries derived from the intensity of light the cube projects on the eye. The successive construction of the state that stands for a red cube is achieved from this representational basis.

Statements by proponents of the inferential account confirm that this is a plausible way of understanding their position. David Marr, for example, writes:

> First, suitable representations are obtained of the changes and structures in the image. This involves things like the detection of intensity changes, the representation and analysis of local geometrical structure, and the detection of illumination effects like light sources, highlights and transparency. The result of this first stage is a representation called

> the primal sketch. Second, a number of processes operate on the primal sketch to derive a representation—still retinocentric—of the geometry of the visible surfaces. This second representation, that of the visible surfaces, is called the 21/2-dimensional (21/2-D) sketch.
>
> (Marr 1982, p. 42)

Andy Clark similarly thinks that Bayesian accounts preserve the idea of perception as proceeding in representational steps from low-level visual areas:

> The representation units that communicate predictions downwards do indeed encode increasingly complex and more abstract features (capturing context and regularities at ever-larger spatial and temporal scales) in the processing levels furthest removed from the raw sensory input. In a very real sense then, much of the standard architecture of increasingly complex feature detection is here retained.
>
> (Clark 2012, pp. 199–200)

In this framework, the visual system reconstructs the layout of a scene by using intermediate sensory states that, at different stages of processing, stand for various elements of both the light hitting the eye (intensity changes) and the world (surfaces). For simplicity, we can call these intermediaries of vision *s-representations* (sensory representations).

This is not the whole story, however. Not every internal transition between representational states in a system is an inference. Associations are transitions between representations that occur merely in virtue of their 'closeness'—or similarity, or some other associative relation.[40] We may suppose that, in many people, the mental transition from the concept SALT to the concept PEPPER occurs by virtue of the fact that the two are often experienced together.[41] Whenever one encounters salt, he or she also encounters pepper, so tokening or thinking one causes tokening or thinking the other. The two are close in our mental space.

The transition between SALT and PEPPER, however, is not inferential. In order to be inferential it would have to be a transition that has some 'logic' to it; that is, it would have to be a transition that is held together by logical relations

40. Mandelbaum unpublished, Sloman 1996, Sperber and Wilson 1987.

41. Following the extant literature, I use small caps to denote concepts. I later use italics to denote non-conceptual representations and tracking states. It should be clear from context when the italics is used to emphasize.

such as entailment, not by mere relations of frequent co-occurrence. PEPPER would have to somehow follow from SALT. Since it presumably doesn't, the move from one to the other is not inferential.

To deem a transition inferential, without appealing to conscious acts of a subject, we can require the transition to be regulated by rules.[42] Rule-regulation makes a transition *logical*, where this does not mean anything particularly positive. The rules that regulate a transition may not be truth-conducive or good in other respects. Transitions governed by 'if you can't beat them, join them' may not be particularly smart or life-preserving. Nevertheless, a transition that is regulated by this rule is inferential. Similarly, if one mentally transitioned from SALT and from SALT IS ALWAYS ACCOMPANIED BY PEPPER to PEPPER, then the transition would be inferential because it would be regulated by a mediating principle (or assumption) that concerns the relationship between salt and pepper. PEPPER would, in this sense, *follow* from SALT.

Inferential transitions typically happen between representations that have linguistic/propositional format—for example, SALT IS ALWAYS ACCOMPANIED BY PEPPER. Indeed it is hard to define such transitions without appeal to a format of this kind. But we should refrain from supposing that linguistically structured representations are required for mental inferences. This is because, when we consider the idea that vision is inferential, the representations involved are not thought to come in linguistic form.[43] The states mediating vision are sometimes presumed to be map-like as in the case of areas of the thalamus, the lateral geniculate nucleus, and the primary cortex which are described as retinotopic 'maps' because they reproduce the pattern of activation of the retina.[44] More often, however, the intermediaries of vision are simply seen as neural states that carry information about environmental elements.

---

42. For the idea of understanding inferences in terms of rule-following—and for some of the problems with this idea—see Boghossian 2008, 2012.

43. See Rock 1983 for the idea that perception is mediated by language-like representations. Interestingly, Pylyshyn also remarks that the indexes in his FINST model can be seen as demonstratives of a language of thought that "allow a person to think about something in the world that was selected in perception" (Pylyshyn 2009, p. 4). I do not pursue the interpretation of Pylyshyn's work on visual indexes here and assume that not everybody is committed to the idea that sensory and perceptual representations have linguistic format. See Palmer 1999, p. 83 for the idea that perceptual intermediaries are not linguistic. Similarly, Bayesian models are inspired by neural networks that do not use syntactic representations.

44. Palmer 1999, p. 155, Purves and Lotto 2003, p. 31; Purves and Lotto 2011, pp. 213–219.

Following these points, we should think of a mental transition as inferential when it is regulated by an encoded principle or an encoded assumption even if the representation that encodes the principle is not linguistic. If the transition from SALT to PEPPER were regulated by an encoded piece of 'knowledge,' as in the aforementioned example, then the move from one to the other would be an inference, even if the knowledge in question is represented in a map-like structure. Similarly, an inferential transition in perception would require that the move from sensory to perceptual representations occurs in virtue of some principles—encoded in some format or other—that comprise the logic of the visual system. If the move from representing the rough boundaries of a cube to representing the cube were regulated by an encoded assumption concerning boundaries and cubical objects, then the transition would be inferential.

Contemporary inferentialists about vision plausibly have this sense of inference in mind. The idea is that there are some heuristic rules encoded in visual systems, and such rules regulate the way percepts are derived from sensory states. Vision science is in the business of discovering precisely what these rules or principles are. For simplicity, we can call these intermediaries of vision *p-representations* (representations of principles).[45]

P-representations regulate the transitions between different s-representations and, in so doing, they constitute a sort of implicit (or, some think, *a priori*) knowledge held by visual systems. Irvin Rock, for example, writes:

> Perception makes use of assumptions and of internalized rules and applies these to novel situations. (. . .) inferences occur on the basis of such rules. 'Rule following' means more than 'lawful'. An object in a free fall follows the law of gravitational attraction, but it does not 'know' any law. Perception, on the other hand—or any mental or behavioral act for that matter—that is based on a rule implies that some lawful relation is 'known' or internally represented.
>
> (Rock 1983, p. 15)

Along similar lines, Simon Ullman holds that perceptual systems are different from systems that merely resonate to environmental properties,

45. Following proponents of inferential accounts and for terminological variance, I use 'encoding a principle (a rule, an assumption)' and 'representing a principle (a rule, an assumption)' interchangeably. By 'encoding' I do not mean anything less committal than 'representing.'

because some 'rules of formation' are 'incorporated' within perceptual systems.[46] Appeal to the incorporated rules explains what the systems do. In non-perceptual systems, by contrast, appeal to physiology and anatomy is enough. David Marr similarly hypothesizes that 'physical constraints' are encoded "in the perceptual machinery."[47]

While in bottom-up approaches to vision the encoded principles serve as premises in perceptual inferences, in top-down accounts they play a different role. They are assumptions that have the primary function of assigning probability. They select what hypothesis concerning the distal environment is initially more plausible—these are the 'priors.' They also indicate which is more plausible given the evidence—these are the 'likelihoods.' As in bottom-up versions, the priors and likelihoods are said to constitute a sort of (*a priori*) knowledge.[48] This knowledge allows the visual apparatus to select percepts on the basis of sensory data (or sensory 'evidence').

In all inferential accounts, an encoded principle or assumption is loosely identified with a piece of knowledge. The identification of 'representing' with knowing is fairly common in psychology, where any contentful state of a system that encodes information about the world, and that is used in a cognitive activity, is thereby deemed a piece of knowledge. From a philosophical point of view this identification is problematic because representing the world to be a certain way is at most only a necessary and not a sufficient condition for knowing. Many think that a representation must also be true and justified in order to constitute knowledge.[49]

---

46. Ullman 1980, pp. 11–12.

47. Marr 1982, p. 219. Marr's book has been the center of a lot of interpretative literature (see for instance Burge 1979, Segal 1989). It is a matter of debate whether Marr held a genuine inferential view of visual perception. Under a plausible interpretation of his work he did not, since, for one thing, he describes the assumptions that regulate visual processing as 'physical constraints.' This suggests that such constraints are physical rather than representational features of the visual system. The correct interpretation of Marr's position, however, is outside the scope of this book. It will not be the focus of much discussion here. What is important is that bottom-up proponents of inferential accounts of vision seem committed to the view that visual systems encode some principles of inference, and this is part of what makes the systems inferential.

48. See Mamassian et al. 2002, p. 13 and Howhy et al. 2008. What makes vision a Bayesian observer is not just that it acts *as if* it is Bayesian, but that it has access to "separate representations of gain, likelihood, and prior" (Maloney and Mamassian 2009, p. 150).

49. See Machery 2009, p. 8 and Karmiloff-Smith 1986. Irvin Rock writes:

> The very essence of intelligence in living creatures (. . .) is the capacity to know, to represent objects, events and relations in a form that is subject to confirmation and disconfirmation.
>
> (Rock 1983, p. 15)

Nevertheless, we can take the identification of knowing with representing to just mean that a system encodes information about the world and that such encoding plays a role in explaining the system's performance. The encoded information need not be available to awareness. There is a question concerning whether this information is innate or acquired.[50] It is widely believed, however, that the information is represented *implicitly*. It comprises a number of tacit assumptions that are not stated in linguistic format and that are not something of which the subject is aware.[51]

Along similar clarificatory lines, visual processing may be inferential but the inferences are different from the ones that, say, Sherlock Holmes performs.[52] Typical rule-following systems are systems capable of entertaining a rule in thought and then conforming to it. In doing so, they are relatively slow and they have some measure of control. Vision by contrast is fast, automatic, and not subject to control. It happens below the conscious level and it is likely subpersonal. It is carried out by relatively independent subsystems of a whole perceiver.

Some proponents of inferentialism think that visual processing is *modular*, having all of the features just listed and additionally being isolated from the influence of background beliefs. Deniers of modularity suppose, instead, that vision is penetrable. Inferentialists all agree, however, that vision resembles Holmes *just* in the sense of operating in a regimented fashion over contentful states.

To make the inferential idea intuitive we can appeal—like inferentialists often do—to the analogy with classical digital computers. Computations are traditionally understood as operations on representations in virtue of rules provided by an algorithm.[53] As such, computational operations are

---

50. Parks and Rock 2000, Rescorla forthcoming, von Helmholtz 1924/2005. Those who speak of the information as being 'a priori' tend to favor the view that the information is innate.

51. Similarly, speakers of a language are said to unconsciously represent and follow some general rules of grammar and this explains how they acquire the language that they speak. Chomsky 1959, 1980. See also Palmer 1999; Pylyshyn 1984; Segal 1989, p. 193 n. 6 and Stich and Nichols 1992 for other examples of implicit knowledge. I discuss the notion of implicit representation further in section 3.2.

52. For the Holmes analogy see Fodor 1984 and 1988. For the differences see Fodor 1988, Gregory 1970, Rock 1983, 1997, p. xiii.

53. Fodor 1975, Pylyshyn 1984, p. xvi. Indeed, though this is no longer the consensus, encoding some rules of processing was once taken to be the hallmark of computational systems (more on this issue in chapter 5). Jerry Fodor famously says:

> A—by now—chestnut of a question that is supposed to embarrass information flow psychologists goes like this: 'If you are willing to attribute regularities in the behavior

inferential even though the inferences are performed in a fast, automatic, and subpersonal way and the computer does not *know*, in any robust sense of the term, what its own rules of processing are. The rules constitute knowledge *in* the system without being knowledge *to* the system. A central idea of the inferential view is that visual processes issue percepts in a similar way to how traditional digital computers issue their output: they manipulate representational states comprising both s- and p-representations.

Of course, not all cognitive theories of perception need to be as committal as inferentialism. Although, for reasons that are somewhat mysterious to me, the visual process is not often described as an association, one could hold that perceiving is mediated by representations but that the transition between them is not regimented by encoded rules.[54] In my terminology, one can hold that perception is only mediated by s-representations.

How robust cognitive positions of this kind are, further depends on how committal an account of representation one holds. The richer a notion one adopts, the more robust a cognitive account will correspondingly be. But leaving this issue aside, we can worry about the next question, which is why vision scientists think that it is necessary to understand vision in this way.

Why inferences? The inverse problem

The claim that perceptual systems perform inferential operations is often introduced by the consideration that there is a one-to-many correspondence between retinal images and their causes. This is sometimes called the 'inverse problem' or the 'underdetermination problem.' The stimulus that hits the retina in the form of a pattern of light underdetermines its causes, in the sense that it is compatible with a number (a large number) of different objects and scenes.

---

of organisms to rules that they unconsciously follow, why don't you say (e.g.) that the planets 'follow' Kepler's laws in pursuit of their orbits about the sun?' The point, of course, is to suggest that the only real case of rule following is conscious rule following by articulate organisms. What other organisms do is (not follow rules but) merely act in accordance with them. It should now be clear how this sort of question is to be dealt with. What distinguishes what organisms do from what the planets do is that a representation of the rules they follow constitutes one of the causal determinants of their behavior. So far as we know, however, this is not true of the planets: At no point in a causal account of their turnings does one advert to a structure which encodes Kepler's laws and causes them to turn. The planets might have worked that way, but the astronomers assure us that they do not. So the solar system is not a computational system, but you and I, for all we now know, may be.

(Fodor 1975, p. 74 n. 15)

54. Dual-process theorists may be particularly sympathetic to this view. See Sloman 1996.

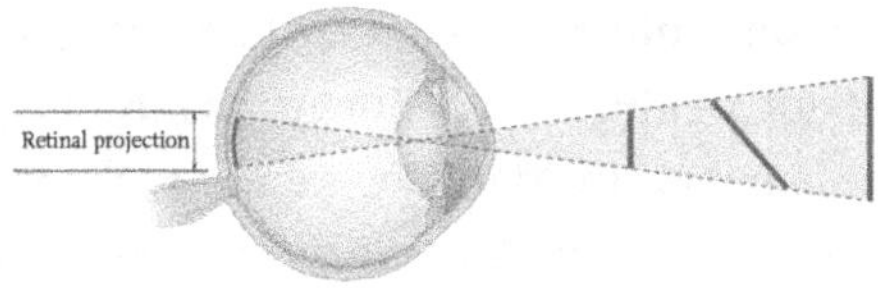

FIGURE 1.1 The inverse problem: retinal projection compatible with different distal causes. From Purves and Lotto 2011, p. 92.

Figure 1.1 illustrates this point. The same retinal projection is compatible with distal causes of different sizes and different orientations, and at different distances from the observer. The visual system has to figure out how to derive a single percept from this ambiguous input.

The system does it by using basic sensory representations and a number of encoded assumptions that constrain how to process the initial stimulation. In figure 1.1, for example, the system may assume that the distal cause is vertical, betraying implicit knowledge of a possible preponderance of vertical structure in the environment. This knowledge rules out certain distal conditions in favor of others and, given enough of it, it guarantees a single, stable percept.

For a further, simplified, example that I use several times throughout the book, think of discontinuities in light intensity at the retina. Such discontinuities can be caused by a number of things in the world, such as edges, cracks, shadows, lines, and changes in color. Correspondingly, the stimulus given by the discontinuities is compatible with a number of different perceptions of the world. We tend to perceive a stable environment, however: we tend to see stable edges rather than changing lines and shadows, when exposed to light discontinuities.

How do we explain this fact? The most natural way to explain it is to suppose that the visual apparatus processes the stimulus by performing something akin to an interpretation. In bottom-up accounts, vision first represents light discontinuities at the retina and then uses some encoded assumptions to process the initial representation. In this case, the system infers the presence of edges by using knowledge that discontinuities of a certain intensity and orientation are typically caused by edges. This is a partial and simplified rendition of David Marr's 'spatial coincidence assumption.'[55]

Since the encoded principles help reduce the possible interpretations of the sensory data, they are described as 'constraints.' Such constraints do not

55. Marr and Hildreth 1980, p. 202. See also section 3.7 for a full formulation of the spatial coincidence assumption. Discontinuities in light intensity in Marr and others are often called 'zero-crossings.'

concern only light discontinuities and edges. At later stages of visual processing, they may be about rigidity, three-dimensionality, shape, surfaces, and a number of other elements. In Marr, for example, the visual process proceeds inferentially until it outputs an object-centered representation of the abstract shape of objects in three dimensions.[56] Others think that perceptual representations have richer contents than what Marr proposes.[57] Bottom-up inferentialists all agree, however, that the output representations are the product of a process that employs constraints.[58]

In top-down accounts, an inference is similarly required to solve the underdetermination problem, but the inference goes in the other direction. The visual system starts by entertaining certain initial hypotheses concerning the distal layout. One sample hypothesis may be that edges are present. Another may be that shadows are present. The system assigns initial probability to these hypotheses by using some encoded principles concerning which hypothesis is more probable to begin with. To do this, vision uses prior assumptions, both concerning the environment in general—for example, the prior assumption that light comes from above—[59] and concerning specific environmental entities—for example, the assumption that edges are very common in our environment (perhaps more common than shadows). The assumptions concerning general environmental facts are called 'hyperpriors,' while those concerning more specific objects and properties are called 'priors.'

---

56. There may be space to disagree with this interpretation (see Prinz 2012). Some passages in Marr suggest that he thought of vision proper as ending with the '21/2-D sketch' (see Marr 1982, p. 268). The exegesis of Marr, however, is not of central importance here. What is relevant is the idea that the visual system proceeds inferentially until it outputs representations that are useful to guide action and that are made available to higher thought.

57. Fodor 1983, pp. 93–94.

58. There are many passages that concern this point (see, for example, Pylyshyn 1999, p. 353, Marr 1982, pp. 219). Here is one lengthy quotation from Stephen Palmer:

> For every 2-D image on the back of our eyes, there are infinitely many distinct 3-D environments that could have given rise to it. (. . .) How does [the visual system] solve this seemingly insoluble problem? Different theorists have taken different approaches (. . .), but the dominant one is to assume that 3-D perception results from the visual system making lots of highly plausible assumptions about the nature of the environment and the conditions under which it is viewed. These assumptions constrain the inverse problem enough to make it solvable most of the time.
>
> (Palmer 1999, p. 23)

59. Ramachandran 1988, Stone 2011, Stone and Pascalis 2010. Strictly speaking, the assumption is that light comes from above and slightly *to the left*, but I leave this complication aside in this preliminary chapter.

So despite the ambiguity of the sensory data, vision forms some probable hypotheses that concern the causes of the data. The hypothesis with the highest prior probability, as determined by priors, is checked against the sensory evidence. The visual apparatus also 'knows' how likely the hypothesis in question is given the evidence (this is the 'likelihood'). As a result, the hypothesis is either confirmed or rejected in favor of a different hypothesis. In Bayesian models this process is sometimes described in terms of the initial hypothesis issuing 'predictions' concerning what the sensory data should be. Predecessors of Bayesian accounts describe this process as involving a 'decision' concerning the more likely causes of the sensory input.[60]

An inferentialist account of vision is perceived to be the only way to solve the underdetermination problem and to account for stability. So vision is inferential in the sense of using representational structures to interpret underdetermined sensation.

This is the type of view that I reject in what follows. I argue that we have a better way of understanding visual processing that explains the relevant performance without appeal to an inference, and to representational structures.

Before I move on to sketch the argument for this alternative, I should note that the foregoing rendition of the inferential view is simplified in several respects, and seeing why this is the case helps clarify a number of important points concerning visual processing. For one thing, the input to the visual system consists of more than just retinal stimuli. The vestibular system,

---

60. This rendition of Bayesian accounts of perception is simplified in several respects. For a more thorough treatment, see section 2.4. Here is a small sample of quotes from proponents of this kind of view. Hohwy et al. write:

> For example, if the hypothesis is that visual input is caused by a box, then it is possible to predict, on the basis of that hypothesis, what the input is going to be as one moves around it. If the prediction turns out to be right, and if the presence of a box is otherwise probable, then the probability for the hypothesis that it is a box goes up. If there are no better hypotheses in play, then this hypothesis wins and the perceptual inference will be that the environmental cause is indeed a box.
>
> (Hohwy et al. 2008, pp. 2–3)

Richard Gregory says:

> At this point we might be tempted into thinking that perception is simply a matter of combining activity from various pattern-detecting systems, to build up neural descriptions of surrounding objects. But perception cannot be anything like as simple, if only because of a basic problem confronting the perceptual brain the ambiguity of sensory data. The same data can always mean any of several alternative objects. But we experience but one, and generally correctly. Clearly there is more to it than the putting together of neurally represented patterns to build perceptions, for decisions are required. (...) The problem is acute because any two-dimensional image could represent an infinity of possible three-dimensional shapes.
>
> (Gregory 1970, p. 25)

for example, provides data that aid the visual apparatus in representing the orientation of distal objects.[61]

There are also general questions concerning the independence of visual processing from the processing of other modalities. The issues pertaining to these questions are not always addressed by inferentialists. They are also neglected in this book where I operate under the idealization that the reconstruction of visual objects occurs somewhat independently of the influence of other sensory modalities.[62]

Additionally, the study of neural pathways suggests that there are two kinds of visual perception, one primarily involved in the guidance of action, and the other primarily involved in recognition—thus primarily involved in rendering the shape of objects.[63] The former is localized in the so-called dorsal stream in cortical areas leading from primary visual cortex to the posterior parietal areas and the latter localized in the 'ventral stream' in cortical areas leading from V1 to infero-temporal cortex. The ventral stream is also said to be responsible for conscious perception.[64]

The models described previously do not always make reference to this difference. They are primarily concerned with the cascade of processes that reconstruct shape and are ultimately used in object recognition (mostly ventral stream processing). This is also the primary subject of this book. There are interesting questions concerning the relationship between the two visual streams and how to understand their interaction.[65] Although this topic deserves further attention, it will not be the focus here. Little is said about how (if at all) the products of the ventral stream interact with the products of the dorsal one, or whether the states produced by the dorsal stream are representations.

---

61. This is why a vertical line is perceived as vertical whether or not our head is bent. The light that the line projects on our retinas is different depending on the head's inclination, but the vestibular system adjusts for this difference (Burge 2010, p. 413, Pylyshyn 1999.)

62. For a discussion of the often pernicious effects of this idealization, see O'Callaghan 2007 and forthcoming. I think that what I say about representation and processing in vision can apply to other modalities. I hope that it also transfers relatively smoothly to multi-modal perception. But I do not pursue the task of showing that this is the case in the present book.

63. Milner and Goodale 1995.

64. Clark 2001, Prinz 2000.

65. Brogaard 2011, Chemero 2009, Mandik 2005, Matthen 2005, O'Regan and Noë 2001. The idea of 'pushmi-pullyu' representations in Millikan 1995 also reflects the effort to understand the ways in which perception and action are linked. On this topic, see also Ballard 1991.

One reason for focusing on the processes involved in object reconstruction is that these processes are more often thought to require the mediation of representational states.[66] Non-representational approaches can be seen as better at explaining perception for action, but representational and computational outlooks are said to be needed for making sense of how vision reconstructs the shape, size, and superficial properties of objects. My aim is to show that, even in this type of processing, we do not need—and are not justified—to appeal to representations.

Summarizing: in inferential models, vision reconstructs representational outputs by using further representations. This ensures the stability of our visual world. Such stability is, by contrast, somewhat of a mystery in direct accounts of perception that allow no inferences. Since the stimulus is ambiguous, our direct perceptions should also be ambiguous. That this is not the case lends support to inferentialism. Vision is then inferential because it is not just involved in *producing* representations, but also because it *presupposes* representations of two different kinds: s- and p-representations. It is a cognitive process in a fairly robust sense.

Associationists hold a less committal view since they only need to posit s-representations. Associationism, however, still counts as a cognitive account. 'Cognitive,' as I intend it, just means 'using representations' and 'cognitive resources' are just 'representational resources.'

It could be, of course, that no system is truly cognitive. If eliminativism about representation is right, this will turn out to be the case. The point here, however, is not whether there are any cognitive systems. The point is rather that, if they exist, explaining what they do requires appeal to the distinctive psychological notion of mental representation.

In what follows, I try to keep inferentialism and cognitivism separate, referring to the former as a subset of cognitive accounts. However, I raise considerations that put both into question. I think that, in many paradigmatic cases, we do not need to, and should not, appeal to any representational structures to explain how percepts are produced. We can think of whatever resources vision needs as functional resources that developed in response to environmental pressure.

I then identified the kind of subject-centered view that I put into question. The view is subject-centered because in explaining vision it appeals to the internal representational resources of observers. The structure of the environment that surrounds us is, of course, very important to establish which

66. Chemero 2009, p. 40, Norman 2002.

resources are encoded within us.[67] But it is because of the resources themselves that we see as we do. Before I present an alternative, I want to conclude this chapter by clarifying what the main argument is, and by placing this project in context.

1.3 The argument

The main argument of this book is that vision is better understood as an embedded system. Appeal to mental representations to explain visual activity is not needed and not justified, save for the outputs of such activity.

I first argue for this claim by noting that the elements that we need to introduce in order to explain the way vision operates are better seen as functional states and features of the perceptual system that are not representations. In particular, I propose to frame p-representations as *mere* biases or constraints—that is, as physical features of the perceptual apparatus that developed under evolutionary and ongoing pressure to perform a certain function. Biases and constraints developed to make the visual system process the input in a certain way. We lack reasons to see such biases as representations in any sense: they are not linguistic, map-like, index-like, implicit, or explicit pieces of knowledge.

I propose further to frame s-representations as states that merely track the environment without representing it, thereby also proposing a distinction between representations and states that are mere reliable mediators. Like biases, tracking states are functional states. They are states that are identifiable by what they do in a system and they help explain its performance. Tracking states are primarily active within a restricted domain (e.g., visual processing) and they figure in subpersonal transitions by responding reliably to some element. It is unclear whether this capacity to respond is enough to give tracking states some type of *content*. There is substantial disagreement on this issue, and some considerations stand against thinking of tracking states as genuinely contentful.[68] I propose to leave this disagreement aside, however, and focus, instead, on other features of tracking states that suggest that they are not representations.

While tracking states are active in a subpersonal transition, they do not also inform person-level behavior in a way that would justify representational status. Additionally, such states are not properly *de-coupled* from their causal and

67. Segal 1989, p. 192.

68. More on this issue in chapter 3. See also Burge 2010, ch. 8.

statistical correlates. They do not have independence from what co-varies with them. Their job is precisely that of responding to their causes and of making something else happen (e.g., by firing). But de-coupleability is precisely one of the essential components of representational states.

De-coupleability is typically understood as a momentary, potential detachment of a tracking state from what causes it to respond.[69] I argue, instead, for a more robust understanding of this notion. Representations are introduced to explain behavior described at a certain level, when the behavior is not easily accounted for by making reference to environmental conditions. Environmental conditions can be understood in terms of stimulus conditions. If representations need to be introduced when appeal to stimulus conditions is insufficient, then the 'job description' of a representation is a performance-guiding state which is independent from its causal and statistical antecedents present in the stimulus. This independence is actual and persistent, not momentary and potential.[70]

In chapter 3, I try to make sense of this independence in terms of representations being about something that, strictly speaking, did not cause their tokening. I suggest that this materializes when a state stands for something *absent* or *distal*. When an internal structure stands for something absent, it stands for something that does not impinge on the senses (e.g., on the retina), and it is de-coupled from its origin. In the usual perceptual condition, for example, an observer may see a whole three-dimensional cube while being exposed only to a fraction of the cube. In this case, the observer is in a state that stands for something that is, strictly speaking, not present to her senses, because the cube does not impinge on them in its entirety. As a result, it is useful to think of the observer as representing because we would have trouble making sense of her behavior in terms of tracking.

Similarly, in seeing a persistent cube, the observer is in a state that stands for what is *distal*—that is, abstracted and removed from the continuous variation of the light that the cube reflects and that hits the eye. Distal properties are properties of objects and events that remain constant despite variation in viewing conditions. A state that stands for them is a state that is removed from its proximal causes. Again, it is useful to see a state of this kind as a representation because it helps us make sense of person-level performance that would be puzzling if we just focused on the stimulus.

69. Chemero 2009, Clark 1997 and Grush 1997.

70. See Ramsey 2007 for the useful metaphor of a job description for representations. See Pylyshyn 1984, p. 12 and Sabo unpublished for the importance of stimulus-independence in relation to psychological postulates.

This characterization gives us a sense of why s-representations hardly qualify as representations. In many cases, intermediary visual states are active only within a restricted domain and they stand for neither something absent nor something distal. They track light frequencies or other proximal conditions. They are not performance-guiding states that are detached from their correlates. We should indeed resist the deflationary tendency of thinking of them as representations simply because they have the function of responding to external conditions. Doing so would result in holding an overly liberal idea of what representations are. Many systems that employ no representations—for example, the immune system—have states that track the environment. That is, they have states that have the function of responding and carrying information about external variables without being representations.

This characterization of representational states also makes sense of why it is plausible to suppose that the products of visual processing are representations, a point that I also addressed in the previous section. When people perceive, they seem to be in states that guide behavior and that have a certain type of *distance* from proximal causes. The states are often about something distal and/or absent.[71] When we see complete, persisting objects, we display representational abilities. Similarly, when we are guided by misperceptions, we exhibit behavior that is explainable if we appeal to what we represent rather than to what is present.

Unlike their sensory antecedents, visual percepts have distinctive representational characteristics. They, of course, may also share a number of similarities with sensory states. We saw that they need not be conscious, have linguistic form, or have conceptual constituents. These properties of visual percepts may raise further questions concerning their ability to play a justificatory or epistemic function. We quite clearly need a story of how percepts that might be unconscious and non-conceptual make contact with beliefs and judgments and can serve to justify them. This should not prevent us from thinking of them in representational terms, however. Given some plausible sense of what representations are, perceptual states qualify.

My argument is then that, if we reflect on the notion of representation and on its evidentiary standards, we can provide a good, and empirically sound, explanation of vision without appealing to representations. In this framework, whether EV is right is partly an empirical issue: it depends on what we need to posit to explain visual competences.

71. A number of non-human animals also exhibit similar perceptual capacities. See chapter 4.

Accordingly, the main argument is *not* that inferential and cognitive accounts are implausible or incoherent. I do not suppose that there is a tension in the idea of a subpersonal system performing inferential operations on representations. On the contrary, I think that this is a good research hypothesis which is supported by some computational systems. In this respect, the argument proposed in this book differs from ordinary-language arguments, or from arguments based on purely conceptual considerations—for instance, arguments based on the appropriateness or inappropriateness of applying psychological concepts to subsystems of a full psychological agent.[72]

The claim that this book defends is thus not that vision couldn't possibly be a cognitive process, or that thinking of it that way is counterintuitive. The claim is rather that cognitive and inferential accounts are empirical hypotheses and, as such, they can be replaced by more plausible empirical hypotheses. I think that the model I offer is more plausible and better supported by current evidence. But one of the upshots of the book—and one of the questions that remains for future treatments—is precisely that we should find ways to test cognitive views vis-à-vis their competitors. If vision is inferential, and if visual intermediaries are representations, then there should be empirical tests that indicate that they are. In section 4.8, I suggest that cognitive penetrability may be one of these tests, but there may be others. Simple performance is not a particularly good test. The visual system can act *as if* it is inferential or cognitive without being inferential or cognitive in any substantive sense.[73]

Given these considerations, I should also note that the argument presented here is only the beginning of an argument. There are, and may well be, visual phenomena that require a cognitive treatment, and section 4.6 gives some examples of such phenomena. What is important, however, is providing some specific coordinates for judging that a treatment of this kind is necessary.

72. Such arguments can be found, for example, in Wittgenstein 1953, 281, 282–284, and in Bennett and Hacker 2003, ch. 3. Wittgenstein's considerations on rule-following, however, inform the notion of a wired or biased system.

73. Vision scientists working in this area recognize this point. Maloney and Mamassian (2009), for example, try to find ways to test the hypothesis that vision encodes priors. They use a transfer paradigm to do it: because their tests involves a visuo-motor skill, they seem to be testing priors in motor behavior rather than in vision proper. Similarly, Irvin Rock recognizes that because his inferential account is less parsimonious than that of Gibsonian competitors, it has an additional burden of proof (Rock 1983, p. 5). Parsimony, as mentioned by Rock, is not a value in itself, since biological systems may be built in all sorts of messy and redundant ways. It is a value in the sense that a theory that posits representational complexity has to show that we have evidence for it.

Without such coordinates, competing visual accounts are hard to judge, and the precise nature of the disagreement between them is difficult to assess.

The next section sketches some of the consequences of accepting the world-centered account defended here, and it places the current project within recent literature in philosophy and cognitive science. EV is both a type of eliminativism and a type of externalism, and, although generally neglected, it is not new.

1.4 The context and the consequences

It is hard to talk of a field in its entirety. Philosophers and psychologists may disagree concerning pretty much every aspect of perception and of its products. It is also, in general, hard to keep up with the latest trends in both science and philosophy. It seems, however, that the following minimal claim can be made concerning ecological approaches to vision. While they remain somewhat of a minority in cognitive psychology, Gibsonian ideas have had quite a bit of uptake in philosophy of mind. They play a role in the enactive view of perception as well as in work in embodied, embedded, and situated accounts of cognition.[74] The emergence of these ideas reflects a general skepticism about the notion of representation as a useful explanatory posit. This skepticism is also supported by work in dynamics and connectionist networks.[75]

As a result, there are, on the one hand, a number of philosophers who are skeptical of the notion of representation altogether. On the other, cognitive psychologists use it heavily in their models of vision and other mental activities. Because of this dissonance, philosophical theories of perception that make no reference to representation—either as products or as intermediaries—may be criticized for being at odds with the science.[76] By contrast, reflection on the notion of representation and advances in dynamics suggest that cognitive psychologists use the notion too much.[77]

The position defended in this book emerges from this interplay. I try to show that models of vision do not need some of the notions that they use, but I also retain representations as products of perceptual processing. My position

74. Chemero 2009, Clark 1997, McClamrock 1995, Noë 2004, Rowlands 1999, 2006, Thompson 2007, Wilson 2004.

75. Beer 1995, Brooks 1991, Dreyfus 2002, Ramsey 2007, Van Gelder 1995.

76. Tyler Burge uses this type of criticism repeatedly against disjunctivism in Burge, 2008, 2011. See also Rescorla forthcoming, 2012b for a similar type of criticism.

77. Chemero 2009, ch. 3.

can be labeled 'non–inferential representationalism,' but I do not use this label in what follows. This is because 'representationalism' is a term that is already used to pick out too much. In some contexts, it is used to refer to the idea that visual experiences have content.[78] In others, it is used to label the thesis that the phenomenological aspect of experience is identical with (or supervenes on) the content of the experience.[79] The kind of representationalism I defend is just the thesis that perceptual states have the features characteristic of representations, while the states that precede them do not.

This position is a type of eliminativism, but a peculiar type of it for a number of reasons. First, the eliminativism I favor does not eliminate representations entirely from a story of seeing. The products are representational while the intermediaries are not.

Second, the embedded view does not appeal to the notion of syntax, or to the causal *inefficacy* of content, in order to do away with representations.[80] It rather appeals to the need to distinguish some functional states of a system—for example, tracking states—from representational states. Appeal to what the states track, or what they co-vary with, may be part of an explanation of what vision does, without that fact lending support to a representational account of vision.

Third, the embedded view constitutes an explanation at the same level as inferentialism. A common worry for some forms of eliminativism is that they 'switch levels,' in the sense of providing accounts of the implementation of mental functions, rather than competing accounts of the functions themselves. Some forms of eliminativism seem to recommend eliminating not just representations but other functional notions from a story of mental competences.[81] EV, however, is not a story of this kind. Biases and tracking states are functional features that, like representations, can be implemented in various different ways. Appeal to them serves to explain visual competences as described in commonsense terms. When we refer to them, we do not move from a description of vision in folk terms to one in neurological terms. Yet the substantive claim is that biases and tracking states are not representations.

78. Schellenberg 2011.

79. Dretske 1997, Lycan 2006, Tye 1997. See also Orlandi 2011a.

80. Stich 1983. See Rescorla 2014 for a recent critical discussion of the purported inefficacy of content.

81. Churchland 1981 can perhaps be read as proposing this type of position when he criticizes both commonsense psychology and functionalism. Functionalism, according to Churchland, is as reactionary and susceptible to elimination as commonsense beliefs and desires.

Indeed, although the book is primarily centered on visual perception, the focus on vision is a way of getting at the foundational issue of what it means for a system or organism to represent. We need to identify the characteristic features of representations, and the distinctive abilities that come with them. Doing so brings us to recognizing an important juncture in nature between systems that merely respond and systems that represent.

In addition to being a form of eliminativism, the approach defended here is a form of externalism, although different from externalism concerning only content, such as the externalist accounts defended by Burge and Putnam.[82] It is a type of process externalism or 'active externalism' where external elements play a crucial role in shaping and explaining perceptual processes.[83] I do not address the further issue of whether the visual system can be said to *extend* outside the head, but my view is usefully described as a type of embedded view because, in Robert Rupert's helpful characterization, visual processing "depend[s] very heavily, in hitherto unexpected ways, (. . .) on the structure of the external environment in which cognition takes place."[84] My project is, in fact, a direct application to the visual case of some of the insights of the literature on embedded and extended cognition. It shows how, by making reference to external variables, we can stop thinking of a process as an inference.

This has consequences for how we understand the basic task of vision scientists. Rather than thinking of them as discovering the internalized and encoded principles that govern visual operations, we should think of them as discovering the environmental contingencies that shaped the functional structure of visual systems. Studying perception involves, centrally, studying natural environments and the stimuli that they produce.[85]

The embedded view is an intermediary position also when it comes to how it relates to computationalism. Embedded, ecological, and, more generally, anti-representationalist models of perception are often skeptical of computational accounts of mental activity. Gibson himself did not conceive of vision as a computational process and cognitivism can be defended precisely by appeal to the computational idea, since it appears to be the only view that

82. Burge 1979, Putnam 1973.

83. Aydede and Robbins 2009, Clark and Chalmers 1998, McClamrock 1995, Rowlands 1999, Wilson 2004.

84. Rupert 2004, pp. 5–6.

85. Geisler 2008, Geisler et al. 2001, Gibson 1979, Rowlands 1999, ch. 5.

is compatible with it.[86] It is common to think that computation and representation go together; so, if a process does not use representations, it is not computational.

This way of thinking is odd, however, since it is precisely work on non-classical computational systems that inspires many of the insights of the embedded account that I defend here. More generally, reflection on non-classical architectures feeds eliminativist intuitions about mental activity.[87]

Instead of holding an embedded and non-computational view, I question the picture of computation and representation as going together. Recent reflection on the notion of computation recommends that we adopt a more inclusive notion.[88] According to the more inclusive notion, computation does not require representational elements. Instead, it can be defined by appeal to functional organization (Piccinini) or by appeal to structural isomorphism (Chalmers). Adopting these more inclusive models permits understanding embedded visual systems as computational, even if they do not manipulate representational states.

The type of non-inferential yet representational position that I propose in this book is not new. Tyler Burge has recently defended what seems to me to be a version of this view. Burge criticizes accounts that he thinks overintellectualize perception in philosophy. Such accounts presume that perceptual representations are not primitive but derived from others. Burge calls positions of this kind 'Individual Representationalism.'[89] According to individual representationalism, in order to perceptually represent an item objectively—that is, as existing in space and time independently of the observer—the individual has to have psychological resources that are explanatorily more primitive, and from which representation of the physical environment is constructed. Burge thinks that there are two families of this view. According to first-family views, perceptions are built from more elementary psychological states. Among the theories belonging to this camp are sense-data theories, according to which subjects construct perceptions out of sense-data, or appearances. Burge says that this type of position dominated the first half of the last century and was later abandoned in favor of second-family views.

86. Fodor 1975, Ullman 1980.

87. See, among others, Ramsey 2007.

88. See Chalmers 2011, Piccinini 2004, 2007, 2008a, 2008b, 2009, Piccinini and Scarantino 2011.

89. Burge 2010, p. 7, 2009, pp. 288–290.

Second-family views hold that, in order to perceive anything, an individual must supplement the perception with other representational states that provide conditions for the individuation of the objects perceived.[90] Quine's holism, or Davidson's idea that representational capacities require various linguistic competences are, according to Burge, examples of this type of view.

Burge thinks that individual representationalism so described, particularly in its 'second-family' manifestation, dominates contemporary *philosophical* reflection on perception, but that it is not warranted by the *science* of vision. I think, however, that the situation may be the reverse of what Burge supposes. Many contemporary philosophical views of perception, such as the 'enactive approach,' do not overintellectualize perception in Burge's sense. They *underintellectualize* perception by supposing that the notion of representation has no place in it at all. They are anti-intellectualist.

On the other hand, it seems that something like a first-family view is still alive in perceptual psychology, at the very least in its rhetoric.[91] A good portion of the science of vision seems to warrant precisely the kind of position that Burge wants to reject.[92] In Burge's words, cognitive accounts of vision are wrong in claiming that perceptual representations are not primitive but built out of others when it is the other way around. Most of our representations are built out of perceptual representations which are primitive.[93]

Andy Clark also defends a position concerning mental life that is sympathetic to an embedded approach. Clark thinks that while representations are not needed to explain a number of intelligent activities (dynamics is enough), they should be retained in an account of some mental competences.[94]

---

90. Burge 2009, p. 288.

91. There are certain rough analogies between bottom-up inferentialism and sense-data theory. In both accounts percepts are built out of sensory states that are more primitive psychological states, and perception is indirect (Price 1950). There are, however, also substantial differences. In general, contemporary inferentialists are not motivated by epistemological considerations (Fodor 1975, pp. 44–48) and they do not presume that we are aware of sensory states. Sense-data and initial sensory states also differ in that the latter are typically taken to be states that can misrepresent (Fodor 1975, p. 48). Sense-data, by contrast, are often said to be psychological entities, irreducible to anything physical, that are immune to error and that exist in a special inner space. I won't dwell on some of the other differences and similarities in what follows.

92. To be fair, Burge discusses inferential accounts of perception and he rightly points out that perceptual inferences in psychological models of vision are not really to be understood as inferences (Burge 2010, chs. 9 and 10). I propose to explain in detail why they are not.

93. Burge 2010, p. 26.

94. Clark 1997.

Inspired by Clark, Pete Mandik develops a position that he calls 'action-oriented representation,' which differs from other enactive views in retaining the idea that action-oriented perceptual states are representational states.[95]

This action-based account displays a number of similarities with the embedded view. EV is also similar to other instances of enactivism as it does not conceive of vision as an isolated and static process of construction. This affinity is particularly evident in my rendition of multi-stability (see section 4.7), which is understood as stemming from visual search. The similarities are also apparent in the recognition that adequate explanations of visual phenomena come from appealing to the richness of the environmental stimuli to which vision is exposed.

The embedded account, however, is also different from enactive and action-oriented views. It does not rely as heavily on the analogy between vision and action, and it does not commit to their continuity. Almost nothing is said here about actions. Save for the account of multi-stability, this book does not tackle the question of whether and in what ways action contributes to perception, by, say, combining with sensory input to solve or reduce the underdetermination problem. It rather develops the point that, even if we do not appeal to movement, visual operations have been overintellectualized.

Furthermore, the embedded view makes no reference to a central explanatory posit of some enactive approaches: the idea of knowing sensory-motor contingencies.[96] This notion is central to some explanations of visual phenomenology—for example, to the explanation of completion. Roughly, seeing an occluded object as complete consists in knowing what type of actions and movements would uncover it. This notion, however, plays no role in my account.[97]

The plan of this book is then the following: chapter 2 presents the embedded view and argues that it is better compatible with current research on vision when compared with inferential accounts. Chapter 3 defends the distinction between representations and states that merely track, and it offers a characterization of representational states that emerges from reflection on

---

95. Mandik 2005. Mohan Matthen (2005) also develops a view of sensory categorization, and of how it relates to action that is, in some respects, sympathetic to an embedded approach to vision. Expanding on the affinities, however, would take us too far afield.

96. O'Regan and Noë 2001, p. 940.

97. This is partly because I am not as concerned with visual phenomenology, and partly because I am not clear on what knowledge of sensory-motor contingencies amounts to—for example, in what sense, if at all, it is like knowledge of environmental facts employed by cognitive accounts. But I do not discuss this topic further.

their explanatory function. Chapter 4 provides situated accounts of stability, constancy, misperception, visual illusion, completion, and multi-stability, and it shows that cognitive penetrability is compatible with the embedded view. Chapter 5 turns to the notion of computation and discusses it in relation to the situated framework.

As a way of introducing the next chapter, I conclude the present one by briefly discussing what I think is an issue for inferentialism with respect to the inverse problem. This issue was one of the initial motivations for writing this book, as it made me question the need to appeal to representational resources in explaining visual processing. Since we can appeal to the structure of the world, it seemed to me that we could do without much of what inferentialism proposes.

Cognitivism as a solution to the inverse problem?

The present project developed because of my discomfort with how inferentialism 'solves' the inverse problem. Inferential views seem to make an illicit appeal to implicit knowledge when the issue is precisely how we have the (unconscious, non-linguistic) knowledge in the first place. Think of the underdetermination problem in the following terms. The stimulus for vision is ambiguous, in the sense of being compatible with many distal causes. A discontinuity in light intensity at the retina can be caused by a number of environmental conditions. The question is, in a sense, how does the visual system *know* that the discontinuity is caused by an edge, rather than a crack or a shadow? The inferential way of answering this question is essentially to say that the system just knows. The system implicitly *assumes* that the discontinuity is caused by edges. This, however, feels a little bit like cheating because the question is, precisely, how does it know *that*? To stipulate that it just knows seems unsatisfactory.

Of course, inferentialists can respond that the system knows it innately, or that it knows it because it has been exposed to the regularity between discontinuities and edges in the past. But these are also unsatisfactory explanations. The innate response essentially concedes that we do not really know how the visual system knows. Claims about innateness are usually claims that we can't explain, in psychology, how something came to be known.[98] The other response does not explain why the visual system picked up that particular regularity instead of all the other ones that it could have also picked up. After all, if

98. Cowie 1999.

discontinuities have multiple causes, the system could have learned any of the regularities involving them. Indeed this is just another way of formulating the underdetermination problem. Why do we get edges from light discontinuities, rather than shadows, for instance?

We could, instead, appeal to external conditions. This would explain how and why visual systems have the implicit knowledge that they have. Edges may be statistically more common than shadows, or they may be the typical causes of a given retinal configuration, or they may be more important to detect, so much so that organisms pick up on them rather than on something else.

If we can appeal to these external facts in explaining how the visual system knows, however, then why not do this from the get-go? If edges are more common or more typical or more important than other entities, then *that* is why we see them. Our visual system does not need to know about them *in any sense of knowing* in order to produce the percepts that it produces. It can simply be wired by the environmental fact in question to produce states that track edges when exposed to discontinuities.

This is one of the issues that motivated this project. It seems that despite their plausibility, inferential views are not explanatory. They seem blind to what is external to the system—for example, to the fact that the stimulus itself has typical causes. Because of this apparent blindness, they also have a tendency to over intellectualize perceptual processes, and to think that visual systems need internal representational resources.

If you are equally puzzled by cognitive 'solutions' to the inverse problem, then you should be interested in the material to come.

1.5 Conclusion

This chapter clarified the main thesis of this book, which is that vision is not a cognitive system or process. It then sketched the main line of argument for this conclusion. The argument is to the best explanation. The world-centered account that I propose is an explanatory powerful research hypothesis that is empirically and theoretically more plausible than its cognitive competitors. The next chapter outlines this account and shows that it accords well with recent models of vision in cognitive psychology. The rest of the book is devoted to arguing for the plausibility and explanatory power of the account. If the view I propose is right, then we do not see the world the way we do because of a construction. We see it as we do because of how it is.

2

The Embedded View

(. . .) the classical theory has a story about how you get from detected properties of the light to perceived properties of the layout. The story is that you infer the former on the basis of (usually implicit) knowledge of the correlations that connect them. Gibson, clearly, does not like this story, but it is quite unclear how he is going to get along without it.

(FODOR AND PYLYSHYN 1981, p. 166)

You can, no doubt, pick up properties of S1 [properties of the ambient light], and, no doubt, some of the properties of S1 that you can pick up may be correlated with properties of S2 [properties of the distant layout]. But you cannot pick up the property of being correlated with S2, and it is hard to see how the mere existence of such a correlation could have epistemic consequences unless the correlation is mentally represented, e.g. as a premise in a perceptual inference.

(FODOR AND PYLYSHYN 1981, p. 168)

Use of Bayesian Decision Theory as a benchmark model does not imply that human visuomotor processing is in any sense Bayesian inference, even when human performance is close to ideal.

(MALONEY AND MAMASSIAN 2009, p. 148)

2.1 Introduction

The last chapter got us acquainted with the idea that visual percepts are built out of other representational states. This chapter purports to show, by contrast, that appeal to representations in vision is largely unnecessary. The chapter introduces a non-inferential way of understanding perception—the thesis that I call the embedded view or EV—and it discusses where the view stands in relation to current theories in vision science.

I start by differentiating representational states and features of a system from functional states and features. Functional states and features are physical or physiological states and features that play a certain function but that are not representation. Accepting the proposed distinction allows us to see how vision could solve the inverse problem without being cognitive.

The general idea is to shift the focus from internal resources to external structure. Appeal to external conditions does double duty. It explains why the visual apparatus has the functional features that it has—that is, it explains why it is biased or constrained or wired to function as it does—and it ultimately also explains why we perceive as we do. The stimulus for vision is, if properly described, richer than we are inclined to suppose, because it is a stimulus that, in practice, is not massively ambiguous. It has usual, discoverable causes. The account of vision that emerges is embedded and situated. It is a direct account, insofar as percepts are obtained without representational intermediaries.

Section 2.3 argues that the embedded view is compatible with, and supported by, recent developments in vision science. In this section, I present an outlook on vision, called Natural Scene Statistics (NSS), that predicts percepts on the basis of the study of environmental regularities. Section 2.4 establishes two points: the first is that EV is also compatible with those recent accounts that advertise as inferential. I claim, in particular, that although Bayesian models of perception are classified as constructive, this is somewhat problematic. It is problematic both because fans of Bayesian models tend to also favor connectionist and embedded understandings of mental processes[1] and because Bayesian inferences have a number of dissimilarities with traditional bottom-up inferences, where these dissimilarities favor a less intellectualized interpretation.

The second point I argue for in this section is that even if we interpret Bayesianism as a fully inferential position, and we view it as incompatible with EV, we still need to supplement it with the study of environmental contingencies. Bayesian inferences need to be grounded in Natural Scene Statistics to explain how the inverse problem of vision is solved. In and of themselves, Bayesian models only account for diachronic aspects of visual perception. They tell us how a visual percept is maintained over time, and how it is changed as a result of stimulus conditions, but the models fail to tell us how the percept is *formed* in the first place. A complete account of vision requires grounding in NSS.

---

1. Most notably Andy Clark.

2.2 Embedded seeing

To introduce the embedded approach we can reflect on why it is plausible to suppose that vision is representationally mediated. As we saw in the previous chapter, cognitive accounts are introduced in connection with the underdetermination problem. The stimulus for vision is compatible with a number of distal causes, but we see just one, and in general, we see that cause correctly. One way to explain this fact is to suppose that vision has some internal resources that supplement the stimulus. These resources are representational, and they come in the form of both sensory representations and encoded assumptions about the world. The assumptions help the system choose one among many possible distal causes. Depending on how robust a notion of representation one holds, this can then result in a more or less sophisticated understanding of the visual act. If, for example, we think of representations as map-like structures, then visual percepts are produced through the mediation of states isomorphic to both proximal conditions and general facts about the world.

Now, while the tendency to appeal to internal complexity seems justified—as some processing must surely occur between stimuli and perception—the assumption that this complexity must be representational is less warranted. Vision scientists often talk of this complexity in ambivalent terms. Think, first, of the supposed encoded assumptions. These assumptions are sometimes described in terms of encoded principles or rules—what I called, for simplicity, p-representations. Other times they are described in terms of constraints or biases. Similarly, early visual states are sometimes referred to as representations and, other times, as simple detectors. I think that there is a big difference between these two ways of describing the complexity. It is, I now argue, the difference between thinking of a system as using representations and *not* thinking of it that way. Let's start with p-representations and with the conditions for thinking of a functional feature as a representation of this kind, and then move on to s-representations.

Relying on the environment: being biased versus following a rule

If we describe p-representations as biases or constraints, then we can think of them as mere functional features of the visual apparatus that make the apparatus act in a regimented fashion. We should not see these features as representing or as having content, as they are literally just connections, akin to wires or valves, that cause something to happen whenever something else happens. In particular, we should not see them as map- or language-like structures that encode assumptions. Moreover, thinking of them as deflationary representations is a first instance of ascribing representations too liberally.

The distinction between a bias and an encoded assumption can be brought into focus by looking at the difference between two types of systems, one regulated by mere adaptive features and the other regulated by representations. The former are *wired* while the latter are *rule-following* systems.[2] A wired—or 'constrained' or 'biased'—system is a system that, under evolutionary or design pressure, developed features that make it act the way it does. The features do not inform any system of anything. They merely came about, or were built into the system, because of some environmental fact.[3]

By contrast, a rule-following system is a system that acts the way it does by encoding the rules that regulate it. In typical examples, rule-following systems are systems that follow instructions. When you follow a recipe for making pizza, either in your head or on paper, the pizza-making behavior is explained by reference to a rule that you entertain and to which you conform. Appeal to the represented rule as a causal antecedent of your behavior is needed to explain your competence. Such appeal is not needed and not justified in the case of merely biased systems.

Of course, a central question in the philosophy of mind is whether there are any rule-following systems at all—that is, whether there are any systems that act as they do because of some contentful state that they are in. Eliminativists answer in the negative, since, according to them, we can explain behavior, including the behavior of apparent cognizers in non-representational terms. If there are no rule-following systems, however, then inferentialism about perception is false from the start, since all systems—including visual systems—are simply wired. The notion of representation would play no role in explaining what they do.[4]

---

2. Burge 2010, p. 405, Dennett 1991, Dretske 2006, Piccinini 2008a, Pylyshyn, 1984 and 1999, Ramsey 1997, Sabo unpublished, Sellars 1954, Wilson 2004, Wittgenstein 1953.

3. Marr's 'physical constraints' may just be such features (Marr 1982). This is why it is a matter of debate whether Marr's view is a genuine inferential view.

4. There is also a more general question concerning whether rule-following is possible. I will not tackle this question here since, again, if rule-following is not possible then inferentialism about vision would seem to be false from the start. Instead, I am assuming that there are some instances of rule-following and I am interested in understanding whether visual systems are rule-following systems. This involves understanding the conditions under which we can tell that someone or something is following a rule. See Boghossian 2012, Kripke 1982, and Wittgenstein 1953 for some of the conceptual difficulties that surround the notion of rule-following.

Supposing that there are some rule-following systems—and presuming inferentialism to be true—leads us to suppose that the visual system is a rule-following system. Appeal to states that serve to encode rules and that affect visual processing is an essential step in explaining vision.

What I propose, instead, is to think of vision as wired—that is, as set to signal, say, edges when discontinuities in light intensity are present. The visual system is biased in this way because of an environmental contingency that is relevant to us as biological systems, namely, that edges and light discontinuities are highly correlated. We can discover this contingency by sampling a very large number of images of natural scenes. Such analysis reveals that edges are very common in our world and that they cause, at the retina, discontinuities in light intensity with certain specific properties. In principle, the discontinuities are compatible with other causes, but in our world they are not, and we can expect the visual system to be wired accordingly.

Since it is presumably advantageous to detect edges, we can expect the visual apparatus to develop features that allow it to track edges, when exposed to discontinuities. This means that the system developed, say, a direct physical connection between states that pick up on discontinuities and states that signal edges. We should not think of this direct connection as a representation. We can simply appeal to the environmental fact to explain what the system does. We *could*, of course, think of the connection in representational terms, but doing so would not be justified unless we had additional motivations (more on this later). As far as explaining the processing goes, we can think of the connection as a mere bias.

To make clear that wired systems do not encode any principles, we can say that they *rely on environmental facts*. They do what they do because of the facts without representing the facts.[5] Notice that the facts do two things in a wired system. First, they help explain why the system is physically configured as it is—for instance, they explain why there is a direct connection between certain of the system's states. Second, the environmental facts explain what kind of output a wired system is likely to produce. In Fred Dretske's helpful terminology, the facts constitute *explanatory* reasons for why the system acts as it does. They explain why something happens without being represented.[6]

5. Pylyshyn 1999, p. 354.

6. Dretske 2006, p. 168. Justificatory reasons, on the other hand, are given by the way in which facts are represented to be. They are reasons *for* something to happen. Justificatory

Computer science draws the distinction between rule-following and wired systems in a vivid way by making reference to two different types of computers: classical digital computers and connectionist networks.[7] There are many different ways of building computers, but *some* digital computers are built to operate on symbols by following some encoded rules or instructions. Instructions are typically encoded in binary strings that are stored in the memory of the computer and that are realized by a voltage level, or some other state capable of physically affecting the machine.[8] Digital computers of this kind may produce an output—such as a series of symbols—when given an input, by following an encoded rule. The representation of the rule enters into an explanation of what the computer does, and the programmer can change the instruction to make the computer act differently.[9]

Other types of computers, however, can be wired to produce a certain output given the input, where that means that they are organized to act in accordance with an instruction without representing it. Connectionist nets are a famous example of artificial systems that are wired in this sense.[10] Such nets are particularly good examples of wired systems because they do not follow step-by-step rules stored in memory, and they do not have easily identifiable structures that stand for instructions. This feature is, in fact, considered to

reasons are also explanatory, but they explain by making reference to the way things are represented to be.

7. In computer science. wired systems are typically labeled 'hardwired' (see Piccinini 2008a, p. 217), but I refrain from using this label because 'hardwired' is too easily associated with 'immutable.' As I make clear in chapter 3, wired systems can change the way they process information. The fact that they are wired only means that they do not follow rules.

8. Piccinini 2008a, p. 214.

9. Again, there is a question concerning whether the computer acts the way it does because of the encoded rule or because of some of other feature of its internal states—for instance, because of the syntactic features of the states that presumably encode rules. Notoriously, viewing mental processes as computational introduces the problem of the epiphenomenology of the mental (Rescorla 2014). This problem raises the possibility of explaining *all* mental activity without appeal to representational notions. The issue here is not, however, whether there are any genuine rule-following systems. We are assuming that there are some in order to make sense of the view that visual processing is inferential. The idea is rather that *if* there are any rule-following systems, then what is distinctive of them is that—in explaining what they do—we appeal to internal states that have content and that are causally responsible for the systems' behavior. If there aren't any rule-following systems, then I guess our job is much easier since all systems would then be wired.

10. They are also standardly used to exemplify associative systems. See Fodor and Pylyshyn 1988, p. 19 for the relation between connectionism and associationism. See section 1.2 for a brief discussion of associationism.

be a particular advantage of connectionist systems, since they can perform functions for which the programmer does not know the rules.[11]

Networks are sets of interconnected units organized into layers. They can be built and trained in a number of different ways. For our purposes, we can focus here, and in the rest of the book, on simple three-layered networks that learn through back-propagation. In networks of this kind, one layer of units receives input from the environment, a second layer produces output to the environment, and a third, hidden, layer communicates only with other elements in the system. Nets can be trained to perform a number of tasks, including perceptual tasks, such as distinguishing underwater mines from rocks given their echoes, recognizing three-dimensional objects from two-dimensional views, and converting written to spoken language.[12]

One way to train networks to perform these tasks is, roughly, as follows. Start with a net whose connection strengths between the units are set at random. Then expose the network to a large number of stimuli—that is, a training set. Finally, adjust the network connections after each individual trial, in order that the network's output would be closer to the desired response if it were exposed to the same input again. This last step is typically labeled 'back propagation.' For example, a mine-detecting network may be exposed to a large number of mine and rock echoes and then adjusted to minimize error—that is, to produce an output that distinguishes mines from rocks by producing different levels of activation of the output units. An algorithm can be written to perform the weight adjustment, but the algorithm only concerns how to change the level of activation of the units to reduce error. It does not consist in a set of assumptions about the environmental causes of mine and rock echoes.

After this sort of training, which consists mainly of weight adjustments, networks are typically able to 'generalize'—that is, to tell mines from rocks, not only in the training set but also in novel instances that weren't encountered during the training period.[13]

---

11. Churchland 1990.

12. Gorman and Sejnowski 1988, Poggio and Edelmann 1990, Sejnowski and Rosenberg 1987.

13. If you are tempted to suppose that connectionist nets are rule-following because they conform to an algorithm that adjusts their level of activation, then you run the risk of blurring the distinction between rule-following and associative architectures. At the very least, the algorithms used in connectionism do not resemble principles that concern the external world. They are rather mechanisms that simply adjust the strengths and units within a system.

What is relevant for our purposes is that networks that perform these kinds of tasks do not do so by following a procedure where the programmer breaks down into steps what to do at each stage to detect mine echoes. In fact, the programmer has generally little idea of what sonic features distinguish mine from rock echoes. She would be unable to write a classical algorithm for the tasks performed by networks.

More to the point, the programmer is typically not even able to single out a specific location in the network that is responsible for a specific type of processing. There is no localizable structure that can be identified as a specific rule. When the programmer wants to change the way the network responds, she simply adjusts the strengths between the units without knowing, and without *needing* to know, what the strengths stand for.

Now, suppose that we built a connectionist network that, when exposed to discontinuities in light intensity of a certain orientation, produces a signal that an edge is present. The network is likely to need some training to be able to do this, since discontinuities are compatible with many distal causes. The training would consist primarily of exposing the network to many instances of, say, edges and shadows, and then adjusting the weights between the units depending on initial performance. When the network is finally successful, it is a wired system that detects edges. It is a system that somehow picks up on the physical characteristics of edge discontinuities without employing the spatial coincidence assumption—the assumption that, according to Marr, relates discontinuities and edges. If we wanted to look for the spatial coincidence assumption inside the network, we would not know where to look.

Along similar lines, if the network failed to detect edges, we would not be able to localize, within it, the specific connection(s) responsible for the failure. Because of this lack of localization, networks are particularly good examples of wired, adaptive systems. They vividly demonstrate the difference between a system that plausibly performs a function by following a rule—for example, a classical computer—and a system that performs a function without doing so, by simply developing physical connections that make it output the response that we want.

I want to also remark, however, that localizability is not the crucial difference-maker between wired and rule-following architectures. Even if we *were* able to localize a structure—that is, even if we *could* point to a part of the network that developed in response to the need to detect edges—we wouldn't thereby also be justified to think of it as a representation of the spatial coincidence assumption. We would need additional motivations to do so.

Notice first that, as far as the detection of edges goes, we can regard the part that we localize as a mere functional feature; that is, we can regard it as a setting or bias of the system without losing any explanatory power. The network can come to issue the correct output simply by virtue of an adjustment of the weights between the units that, in turn, affects their levels of activation. This, and not what the units and connections supposedly stand for, is what matters for the performance of the network. Again, the programmer does not *need* to know what the connections stand for. All she cares about is that the network outputs the correct response, and she makes that happen by adjusting the weights.

To confirm this point, consider that there are computational systems, such as simple arithmetic logic units, that resemble traditional digital computers more closely than connectionist networks, but that are wired rather than rule-following (more on this in chapter 5). There are computers that, unlike nets, operate over symbolic elements, but that do not execute algorithms. They are simply built to conform to a principle without having any structure—saved in memory or elsewhere—that encodes the principle.

Consider also that there are pretty clear examples of wired systems where we *might* point to a feature that regulates a given function—and where the feature developed in response to environmental pressure—but where such a feature is not a representation. Simple biological systems are a good example.

Ducklings apparently follow the first moving thing they register because that first moving thing is typically their parent, but, plausibly, they do not represent this fact. They have states that react to movement and these states trigger the ducklings' motor system to follow the movement. Yet there is no structure that encodes knowledge of the correlation between movement and parents. Historically, the fact that the first moving thing *is* their parent 'put its stamp' on the system. This means that the environmental fact in question caused a strengthening of the transition between states that track movement and states that cause the ducklings to follow the movement. The fact, and the corresponding principle, however, are not represented internally. Our ability to localize the strengthened transition does not, *per se*, justify ascription of representations.

In a similar vein, some snakes have facial pit organs that are sensitive to radiant heat.[14] This, among other things, allows them to track and capture prey, because the prey's body temperature—for example, that of mice—exceeds the typical environmental temperature. The snakes' facial pit organs are sensitive to prey in virtue of a reliance on the environmental fact that prey typically has body temperature within a certain range. We should not see facial pit organs as encoding this fact, however. The organs simply evolved to signal

14. Churchland and Churchland 1983, Gracheva et al. 2010, Kardong and Mackessey 1991.

the presence of prey when a source with a certain temperature is present and to correspondingly guide the snake's behavior.

For an example that involves artifacts, think of simple fire alarms such as smoke detectors. In general, fire alarms rely on the correlation between smoke and fire. They signal fire when they detect smoke because the two are correlated, without needing to encode the correlation.

Optical smoke detectors rely on additional facts. They are sometimes built to be sensitive to the presence of smoke in the following way. A simple light source produces a beam of light within a relatively small chamber. When smoke enters the chamber, it deflects the beam to a sensor that triggers the alarm. The fact that smoke particles deflect light particles is used to perform the detector's function; it enters into an explanation of how the detector is sensitive to smoke. Nevertheless, nowhere in the optical chamber is the fact encoded. It would be somewhat frivolous to think of the detector as first representing that light has been deflected and then as inferring that smoke is present by using knowledge—in *any* sense of 'knowledge'—that smoke deflects light. The fact correlating smoke to light is simply exploited to allow the detector to do its job.

In all of these cases, we have no reason to think of these different systems as having linguistic or map-like structures that stand for complex environmental facts, such as the relation between smoke particles and light deflection, or between movement and parents, or between heat and prey. We should also resist the tendency to think, in a deflationary spirit, that the strength of the transition between, say, heat-tracking states and movement-producing states is a representation, simply because it is a feature of the system that developed in response to a complex environmental contingency. Thinking of the connection this way is unnecessary and trivializing, as all sorts of systems would then turn out to be rule-following.

If we use a deflationary notion of representation to argue for the representational status of simple functional features, then it seems that we won't be able to draw a distinction between rule-following and wired systems at all, since virtually all biological and organic systems, including plants and other very simple mechanisms have features that evolved in response to environmental pressure—that is, features that lawfully co-vary with some stable worldly fact and that have the function of doing so.[15]

15. Indeed if we just look at causal co-variance then we might have to include even rivers and planets as rule-following systems since they have states—for example, the riverbed—that

Certainly, associative systems—that is, systems that instantiate transitions between internal states that are regulated by closeness or similarity—would be rule-following in this deflated sense, thus also being inferential at base. Associative systems could be said to follow a closeness or similarity rule. Connectionist networks would also be rule-following, since we can point to the whole set of interconnections in a network and say that it must encode some assumption or other. The strengths of the connections in our imaginary edge-detecting network evolved, during the training period, to allow the network to detect edges, so they can be seen as encoding the spatial coincidence assumption. This only shows, however, that if we follow deflationary instincts, we end up blurring the distinction between rule-following and wired architectures, and we trivialize what it is for a system to follow a principle.

The point I am making is hardly controversial. Alleged proponents of deflationary accounts of mental representation, like Jerry Fodor and Fred Dretske, agree that there is a difference between systems that are regulated by encoded principles and systems that are not.[16] So they would presumably also agree that many biological creatures have adaptive features that regiment them without being representations.[17]

Zenon Pylyshyn makes this point explicitly when, in characterizing the computational theory of mind classically understood, he says:

> The requirements of strong equivalence and independent constraints lead us to recognize a fundamental distinction between rule-governed or representation-governed processes and what I call functional architecture. By 'functional architecture' I mean those basic information processing mechanisms of the system for which a non-representational or nonsemantic account is sufficient. The operation of the functional architecture might be explained in physical or biological terms, or it might simply be characterized in functional terms when the relevant biological mechanisms are not known. This particular distinction is crucial to the enterprise of taking the computational view of mind seriously.
>
> (Pylyshyn 1984, p. xvi)

---

lawfully co-vary with the quickest path to the ocean. Thinking of the river as 'knowing' the quickest path to the ocean is a short step from there.

16. See, for example, the quote from Fodor in footnote 53 ch.1.

17. This is perhaps a sign that alleged deflationists in effect hold more robust positions—more on this in section 3.3.

Biases and constrains are functional features of a system that can be realized in various different ways, and they are not representational features. They regiment a system without having content and representing worldly events. My proposal is that vision is a regimented apparatus using functional features of this kind to produce percepts.

Wired or biased systems do not react to the environment at random. In the case of ducklings, they react as they do because the first moving thing is usually their parent, and it is typically advantageous to stay close to one's parent. We can give a perfectly satisfactory explanation of what wired architectures do, however, by simply appealing to functional and environmental facts.

This is an important remark, because the fact that wired systems are not rule-following is not a *mere* intuition. It rather follows from the fact that representational notions are only needed when organic, functional, and environmental conditions are insufficient. Since we can explain the behavior of certain systems without appeal to representations, we should not introduce them. To think of ducklings, snakes, and smoke detectors as encoding assumptions is explanatorily superfluous. It would require additional motivations—that is, motivations that are different from the simple fact that they have a feature (a direct connection) that evolved in response to environmental pressure and that is involved in regimenting a restricted domain of processing.

Cognitivists agree that we would need additional motivations in these cases, and these motivations have to do with explaining agent-level performance.[18] Justified ascription of representation of principles (p-representations) requires quite a bit of evidence, arguably more evidence than what is required for ascribing representations of properties and entities (s-representations). Before we move on to speak of s-representations, it is useful to glance at what these motivations are for the ascription of p-representations.

Signs of rule-following

When is ascription of p-representations justified? One plausible idea, that comes from both computer and cognitive science, is that we could count a principle as represented if the principle were available in different contexts

18. See Pylyshyn 1999 and Maloney and Mamassian. 2009. See also Evans 1981 and Davies 1987 for the more general question of how to empirically ground ascriptions of tacit knowledge—for example, knowledge of grammar.

within the organism—for example, available to higher thought.[19] If a principle showed up, for instance, in the subject's belief set and acted as a justifier for judgments, then we would have some reason to suppose that its representation is stored somewhere and then retrieved for a number of cognitive tasks. In classical digital computers, for example, the principles of processing are stored in memory.

According to this criterion, a system uses p-representations not just when it has an evolved structure that seemingly co-varies with some fairly complex fact, but also when the structure is active in different contexts. In paradigmatic examples of rule-following—for instance, in the case of human cognizers—the principles that regulate a certain system, even when unconscious, often show up in different contexts. The rules that regulate your pizza-making skills, although generally not present to your consciousness, can be retrieved in a number of contexts for justifying beliefs concerning pizzas.[20]

More problematically, implicit assumptions concerning underrepresented social groups—for instance, the assumption that a certain class of people is unreliable—are typically active in a number of decision-making contexts, such as hiring, sitting behavior, and interview selection. These assumptions can be brought to consciousness for justifying discriminatory practices.[21]

In ducklings and snakes, in contrast, the principles regulating their movement seem to only regulate what happens in a very restricted domain. Neither do the principles show up in the belief set, for it is even dubious that ducklings and snakes have beliefs. Similarly, whether visual systems are wired would partly trade on whether the principles that they presumably encode, such as the spatial coincidence assumption, show up in the perceiver's belief set—not, of course, as a result of doing vision science but as a result of simply perceiving.

A second, recognized, symptom of rule-following is that a system is responsive to evidence that runs contrary to its own principles of operation.[22] The thought is that systems that (unconsciously) follow represented rules—for

19. Pylyshyn 1999, pp. 355–356.

20. If you do not have any pizza-making skills, then that is quite tragic. For a good discussion of whether other skills are regulated by rules, see Stanley 2011.

21. Mandelbaum unpublished. Implicit attitudes are overwhelmingly described as implicit *biases*, suggesting that they are not representational features of cognizers. Contrary to this linguistic practice, there is good evidence that implicit attitudes are represented assumptions in good standing, as they can be made explicit, they are active in different contexts, and they appear to be reason-responsive.

22. See Pylyshyn 1999, p. 355.

instance, thinkers—are typically sensitive to incompatibilities and capable of responding to them. If your pizza-making rules are not pizza-conducive in a given context, perhaps due to unusual humidity, you are likely to change the rules and/or to refrain from conforming to them. Your evidence-responsive performance, in this case, indicates that you represent the rules.

By contrast, ducklings follow the first moving thing they register even if they have evidence that the thing is not their parent. They may be surrounded by people and yet they follow the first moving thing anyway. They are not sensitive to the fact that, in a given context, the principle may not be conducive to survival. This does not mean that the ducklings' tendency is completely unchangeable—a point that will be of central importance in explaining the adaptability of vision in later chapters. We could perhaps train ducklings and other organisms that appear to be wired to act differently, but this training involves reinforcement and reward, not the presentation of contrary evidence.[23] Wired systems are not systems whose behavior is immutable—as connectionist networks amply demonstrate. They are systems whose behavior does not change simply by virtue of presenting information that runs contrary to how they are set to function.

Not coincidentally, the idea of being sensitive to contrary evidence is also one of the ways, in psychology, to draw a contrast between associative and rule-following systems. Associative systems instantiate transitions that occur not by virtue of rules but by virtue of some other relation.[24] In a connectionist network, for example, a given level of activation in the hidden units occurs whenever a level of activation is present in the input units because the two are connected.

Inferential systems and associative systems are thought to differ in a number of ways. Transitions within an associative system are generally more durable and more quickly primed than transitions within an inferential system. A difference that is relevant to our present purposes, however, is that associative transitions are not reason-responsive. You cannot throw logic at an association and hope that it will change. If I am conditioned to token PEPPER whenever I token SALT, then pointing out that one does not mean the other will not disrupt the association. When I think of salt, I will automatically also think of pepper. Similarly, if, with the help of food rewards, I condition a

23. Weiskopf 2008 discusses some literature on how to affect imprinting in birds.

24. Many systems we encounter may instantiate a mix of associative and inferential transitions. I simplify here for expository purposes.

pigeon to peck on a key when a certain stimulus is present, then it will not do much to tell the pigeon to stop. Instead, I can either extinguish the association or use counterconditioning, where both of these methods involve changing environmental contingencies.

The idea, then, is that a second source of justification for thinking of a system as rule-following is if the system appears sensitive to contrary evidence. If the visual system is wired, then it should not be responsive to reason and contrary information. I discuss whether this is the case in sections 3.7 and 4.8.

We now have some better sense of how to distinguish wired from rule-following systems. The fact that a system is well-modeled by a connectionist architecture, rather than by a classical one, is preliminarily suggestive that the system is wired. What's more central is whether the system is reason-responsive, and whether the principles it employs are active in a number of contexts. That a system simply has physical features that perform a certain function is not a good reason to count it as rule-following. Indeed, such features may be precisely what make the system biased or constrained.

These criteria may still not be sufficient to decide in dubious cases. Disagreement may remain concerning systems that meet one of these criteria but not the others. Nevertheless, the conditions pick out a real distinction by describing some important differences between clear cases of rule-following and wired arrangements. Importantly, based on the foregoing criteria, whether a system is wired or rule-following is an empirical question, and this question does not just trade on whether a system acts *as if* it is rule-following. Both wired and rule-following systems act as if they perform inferences, but, if our characterization of inference is right, then only the latter genuinely do. The further question is whether vision is wired or rule-following. My present proposal is that it is a wired system.

According to EV, the visual system has physical features that make it act in a lawful manner. We should refrain from thinking of such features as representing anything. The features are biases shaped by environmental contingencies in the evolutionary past *and in the present*, and we can appeal to such contingencies to explain what we see. In the visual system, *discontinuity in light intensity* activates *edges* without conforming to a represented rule. The two states co-activate because of their statistically frequent co-occurrence—that is, because of the statistics of natural scenes where edges are very frequent and cause discontinuities of a certain kind at the retina. Systems that had (and have) a strong connection between the two types of states fared better in the world.

Before we move on to discuss s-representations, let me briefly remark that there is good evidence that the visual apparatus is physically affected and shaped by environmental facts. There are examples that suggest that the visual system has physical features that implement the functional features I have called biases or constraints.

It is *prima facie* plausible to think that the already noted existence (see section 1.2) of two streams of visual processing—one roughly devoted to object recognition and the other to action guidance—reflects the relative independence of what an object is from where it is.[25] The fact that identity and location are independent variables favored the development of different channels for their processing. This fact biased the visual system to process identity and location separately.

Similarly, the ability of neurons to inhibit each other, in what is called 'lateral inhibition,' is connected to the need to be particularly sensitive to light discontinuities given their correlation with important elements in the world, such as edges.[26] An excited neuron exposed to intense light reduces the activity of its already less excited neighbors, exposed to less intense light, thereby heightening our sensitivity to intensity differences. The fact that intensity differences are important shaped, and continues to shape, the visual apparatus to be extra sensitive to them. Lateral inhibition is then a physical feature of our neuorological make-up that performs a certain function—making us sensitive to light discontinuities—without being a representational feature.

Summarizing: if p-representations are constraints, then vision is not rule-following and, therefore, not an inferential system. It may be a cognitive system—an associative one, for instance—but it is not inferential. Whether it is cognitive depends on the further question of whether it is mediated by s-representations. Such representations are sometimes described as detectors, and I want to now suggest that this is an important slip, since mere detectors are not representations at all. We need to draw a distinction—which we already find in different areas of philosophy and cognitive science—between a state that merely tracks, indicates, registers, or responds and a representation. In other words, we need to recognize a distinction between mere sensitivity and representational capacity.[27]

---

25. Thanks to Andy Clark, personal communication, April 25, 2013, for this suggestion.

26. Coren et al. 1999, Von Bekesy 1967.

27. Burge 2010, Cantwell-Smith 1996, Clark and Toribio 1994, Dretske 1991, Fodor 1986 and 1990a, Pylyshyn 1984, Ramsey 2007, Sabo unpublished.

Tracking

Tracking states of a system are states that operate in a very restricted domain—for example, a subpersonal transformation—and that are not de-coupled from their causal origin. They require contact with what they stand for, consequently acting as simple reliable mediators. In William Ramsey's useful terminology, such states are simple relay switches.[28]

Tracking states are often thought to lack genuine content as they resemble biases and constraints in being simple evolved features of a system.[29] Leaving the issue of content aside, however, I think that even if we were willing to concede that, in some minimal sense, tracking states have content—and what they track *is* their content—we should still distinguish them from representations. Representations, in whatever format, typically come with both observable performance-contribution and independence from their correlates, particularly from their *causal* correlates. This is essentially because they are introduced when appeal to what is outside the organism is explanatorily unsatisfactory.

In chapter 3, I spell out the independence of representations from their co-variants in terms of them standing for something absent or distal, where both the notions of 'absence' and 'distance' have something to do with a state detaching from the constantly changing stimulation—such as the light hitting the eye. Something is absent if it does not impinge on the senses, and something is distal if it is a persisting property or entity that abstracts from the continuously changing proximal conditions. Seeing a stable, complete object, despite the fact that not all of it impinges on the senses, and despite the fact that what impinges on the senses is not stable, is a paradigmatic instance of being in a representational state of this kind.

In a recent book, Alva Noë argues that one of the fundamental problems of psychology is the problem of presence.[30] By contrast, I am suggesting here that one of the fundamental issues of psychology is the problem of absence and distance. Paradigmatic psychological notions, such as the notion of mental representation, enter into an explanation of what a system does, when appeal to what is present in the stimulus is not sufficient to understand performance. The presence of a representational mind starts surfacing in an

---

28. Ramsey 2007, p. 126.

29. Burge 2010, ch. 8 argues for this point with respect to what he calls 'registering' states.

30. Noë 2012.

organism when there is independence between what the organism does and what is given to it.[31]

In arguing for a distinction between tracking and representing, I am not advocating an overly demanding notion of representation. I am rather pointing out that some functional states and structures do not meet even minimal conditions for representational status. Although a neuronal state can lawfully co-vary with internal and external parameters—in this sense carrying information about them—it may not serve to represent such parameters. It may simply become active when certain conditions obtain and cause something else to occur. Some cognitivists indeed explicitly agree with this position. Zenon Pylyshyn for example, writes:

> Although certain neural states could be described as representing the state of the retina, the motor system, or some other part of the nervous system (as P.S. Churchland, 1980, does), the relation between the neural state in question and what it is taken to represent fails to meet numerous conditions on representation suggested above; for example, transitions among them cannot be described in terms of such content-dependent rules as inference. These relations are purely causal and must be sharply distinguished from semantic relations.
>
> (Pylyshyn 1984, p. 47)

Similarly, I think that presumed deflationists agree that an internal state of a system may reliably respond to a certain element, and have the function of doing so, without yet being a mental representation—a point on which I will elaborate in section 3.3. They agree that whether the state is a representation depends on further facts—for instance, on whether the state informs higher thought and organism-level behavior (Dretske), and on whether it tracks non-nomic properties (Fodor).

Intermediaries of visual processing either do not contribute to observable performance or they lack the relevant independence from their correlates (or both). Some examples in the visual systems are retinal maps and light discontinuity trackers. Retinal maps are presumably isomorphic to the image projected on the retina, but they are not sufficiently removed from that image, and they do not reproduce something absent. They are rather reliable intermediaries that usefully co-vary with retinal parameters. They adjust continuously

31. In line with this idea, Brentano famously thought that one of the central issues in psychology is to understand how mental states can be about absent entities. Brentano [1874] 2009.

by reacting to what is present. Thinking of them as map-like representations buys us no explanatory advantage.

Similarly, very early stages of visual processing, such as discontinuity detectors, are not representations. They stand for something present and they continuously respond to it. Like states of snakes and ducklings that respond to heat and movement, early visual states respond to the presence of a physical quantity and make something else happen.[32]

Another way to see this point about early vision is by reflecting back on p-representations. In that case, we might have been tempted to think of the evolved features of a system as representations because such features came about in response to some *distal* and fairly complex facts—for instance, that warm things are prey. Indeed, I think that whether a state is about something distal plays a big role in the cognitive scientist's willingness to regard it as a representation. In the case of early visual states, however, we do not have this motivation since they do not stand for anything distal. They simply track what is present.

There are also intermediaries of vision that are somewhat in between retinal maps and percepts—for example, Marr's 21/2 D sketch. I return to their status in section 3.6. I want to now notice two things about them. The first is that, given connectionist models of perceptual activity, it is not clear that we are going to be able to neatly separate different stages of processing that stand for well-defined quantities. If the visual process is well-modeled by connectionist nets, then, although there are intermediate stages to it, these stages may not stand for anything recognizable and constant over time. It is notoriously difficult to figure out what the hidden units in a network stand for, and, more importantly, it is not needed to understand how the network works and how it performs its function.

Second, while these states might have some independence from their correlates, it is far from clear that they affect person-level performance. Intermediate stages are typically thought to only influence visual operations—that is, to be proprietary to vision. Accordingly, in many cases, we may be able to think of them as causal intermediaries that have no representational function with no explanatory loss.

32. I am assuming here, for argument's sake, that we can explain the snake's chasing behavior and the ducklings' movement by appeal to internal functional states that respond to proximal conditions—for example, to movement and heat. This may not be correct. We might need to suppose that these animals have states that stand for the distal causes of the proximal stimuli, in which case they would not simply be stirred by movement and heat. They would represent distal entities.

By contrast, later visual states, the 'outputs' of visual processing, are plausibly representations, because they inform actions that are stimulus-independent. Completion is a paradigmatic example of this (see section 4.6). We avoid or grab objects in the environment because we visually perceive them as complete even if we are exposed only to their fragments. The fragments are what impinge on our senses, but we appear to act based on states that stand for more than just the fragments.

As in the case of p-representations, we should of course be open to thinking of the intermediaries of vision as representational structures if this proved empirically more sound. This, rather than being controversial, is just how it should be. Whether a system employs representational states is partly an empirical question. It depends on what we need to posit in order to make sense of what happens. Accordingly, given the great variety of phenomena investigated by vision scientists, we should be open to the possibility that some visual operations are operations over representations. In some cases, vision may be cognitive. What is important is to have some idea of how to judge that it is.

With the distinction between representational and tracking states under our belt, we can re-introduce the embedded view. According to EV, visual systems are sensitive to certain environmental features—light discontinuities, for instance—and rely on the environment to create representations. Forming perceptual representations does not presuppose the possession of other representational resources. The visual system engages in a good amount of processing where it responds to environmental properties, and the states that respond to such properties have causal effects that depend on how environmental facts wired the system, but this type of processing does not consist in an inference. It does not resemble the operations of intelligent agents. It should not be thought of that way. We can understand what the system does, prior to the production of visual representations, in non-representational terms.[33]

33. Denying that the visual system engages in a process that resembles the processes of intelligent agents does not amount to denying that it is, in some sense, intelligent. Following Gilbert Ryle (Ryle 1949) we may accept that intelligence can be a matter of performance rather than a matter of the causal mechanism that is responsible for the performance. Whether or not something or someone is intelligent is a matter of how adaptable or impressive their performance is when placed in certain circumstances, and not necessarily a matter of whether a ratiomorphic or inferential process precedes the performance. Similarly, the fact that vision is non-cognitive does not imply that it is not 'mental.' Even though representations are distinctive psychological posits, they are not the *only* psychological posits. The set of states and processes that are mental may be larger than the set of states and processes that are representational. Some suppose, for example, that there are states—such as pain—that are mental, having a certain phenomenology, but that do not represent.

I now move on to discuss where EV stands in relation to current developments in vision science. In the next section, I discuss an approach—Natural Scene Statistics—that is explicitly sympathetic to a non-cognitive outlook. In section 2.4, I present, instead, a view—the predictive coding approach, or the Bayesian approach to perception—that is presumably inferential, and I argue for two claims. The first claim is that predictive coding accounts have features that favor a non-inferential and embedded interpretation. The second claim is that, even if we view Bayesian approaches as inferential, we need to integrate them with Natural Scene Statistics to obtain a comprehensive account of vision. The aim of what follows is to start establishing the theoretical and empirical plausibility of EV.

2.3 Natural Scene Statistics

Natural Scene Statistics is an approach that originates in physics[34] and that enjoyed some recent development due, in part, to the improved ability of computers to parse and analyze images of natural scenes. NSS comes in different forms. Some of its practitioners are sympathetic to inferential accounts of perception and accept the statistics approach together with Bayesian ideal observer theory,[35] while others are critical of Bayesian outlooks.[36] I briefly describe this disagreement at the end of this section, but, first, I want to outline the features of the approach that are relevant to the embedded view. NSS is a highly technical field that employs notions from physics and mathematics and I do not presume to understand it in full detail. In what follows, I try to capture the features of the view that are particularly relevant to the inverse problem.

One of the fundamental ideas of NSS is to use statistical tools to study *not* what goes on inside the head, but rather what goes on outside—for example, what are the likely environmental causes of retinal images. NSS is interested both in what is more likely present in the environment or, more tractably, in how probable a given cause is, and in the relationship between what is in the world and the stimulus it produces.

Researchers in this paradigm often tackle the first problem—that of finding what is more likely present in the world—by taking a physical object or property and measuring it in a large number of images of natural scenes. Both macro and micro objects and properties can be the object of such analysis. We can

34. Geisler 2008 p. 169.

35. Geisler 2008. More on this in section 2.4.

36. Howe et al. 2006, Yang and Purves 2004.

calculate the incidence of a certain luminance in natural environments,[37] or the incidence and characteristics of edges in the environment.[38] In doing this, we trust that the sample of images of natural scenes that we use are representative of the natural world at large (figure 2.2 gives an example of one such image).

When we proceed in this way, we discover facts about the world that are not entirely transparent to the naïve observer. Controlling for distance and direction relative to one another, for example, we may find that edges are overall more likely to have a parallel orientation or to be parallel.[39] This suggests that there is a great deal of parallel structure in natural images, and hence in the world, which may be due to growth, erosion, shading, and other factors. In the context of perception, we may further presume that this fact had an influence on the visual system by wiring it to prefer parallel structure. In other words, we can explain why vision developed a bias for parallelism. Such a bias is in place because of environmental contingencies. Given this bias, it would be unsurprising if we were to see edges as parallel even if their retinal projection is compatible with other distal configurations.

In addition to calculating what is common in the world, proponents of NSS can also, by using similar methods, calculate the kind of input that environmental elements project on the retina. This is typically done by measuring the probability of a given retinal stimulation being caused by a particular item. So, again, we may consider edge 'elements' in natural images. Given what we know about the receptive properties of the retina we can select, in natural scenes, the elements that are likely to cause a zero-crossing—that is, a significant change in intensity as picked up by retinal receptors. By so doing, we identify edge or contour elements in natural scenes and the type of projection that they are likely to produce. We can then study what properties the edge elements have in our environment and what properties they are likely to have at the retina. We may find, for instance, that for any two edge elements and for all distances, if the elements are oriented more or less in the same way then they are more likely to be co-circular—that is, tangents of the same moderately sized circle. This reflects the fact that natural contours have relatively smooth shapes.

This fact helps us predict what perceivers see. Edge elements that are co-circular are more likely to come from the same physical edge.[40]

37. Howe et al. 2006, Yang and Purves 2004.

38. Geisler et al. 2001.

39. Geisler et al. 2001, p. 713.

40. Geisler 2008, p. 178.

By calculating what type of projection the oriented elements produce on the retina, we can predict whether any two elements will be seen as belonging to the same physical contour. In other words, given what we know about the world and about retinal capabilities, we can get a sense of how *likely* it is that a particular retinal configuration is caused by a single physical edge. With this knowledge in hand, we predict what observers see.[41]

In this framework, we do not hypothesize that a retinal projection gives rise to the perception of a single contour because of an inference. We rather accept that we see edge elements as continuous because this configuration is the most likely cause of a given retinal state. The stimulus for vision, although ambiguous in principle, is not ambiguous in our environment, and, unsurprisingly, we are equipped to be sensitive to this fact. Accordingly, prior 'experience' makes a difference to how we see the world. If we understand 'experience' as prior exposure—rather than as perceptual experience—then a visual system that is repeatedly exposed to certain environmental regularities is likely to develop features that favor certain percepts. This restricts the inverse problem enough to make it solvable.

A more detailed example may further clarify this way of approaching vision. This example concerns the perception of brightness—that is, the perception of how light something is—and it aptly demonstrates how appeal to environmental contingencies can help make sense of what we see.

Brightness perception in NSS

The intensity of light reflecting from objects in the spectrum that our eyes are able to respond to is typically called 'luminance.'[42] Luminance is a physical quantity measurable in natural scenes. An increase in luminance means an increase in the number of photons captured by photoreceptors and an increase in their levels of activation.

We may intuitively suppose that the perception of brightness—that is, how bright or light we perceive something to be—is a direct measure of luminance. This, however, is famously not true. Target patches that are equi-luminant appear different in brightness depending on context. In figure 2.1 the target

41. Or we first apply a gain/loss function and then issue the prediction. Like in Bayesian models of perception that I discuss in the next section, different proponents of NSS use different methods to issue predictions. This point will be relevant later when I describe and assess the claims of empirical ranking theory.

42. Purves and Lotto 2003, ch. 3.

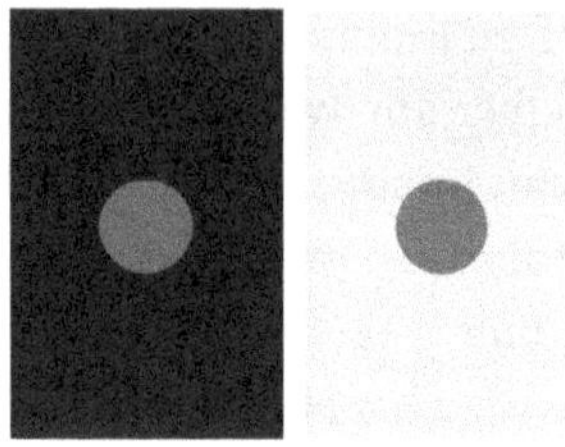

FIGURE 2.1 Brightness contrast effect. From Purves and Lotto 2003, p. 56.

dot with lighter surround appears darker than the equi-luminant target dot with darker surround.

Luminance and brightness perception are not directly proportional because, in natural environments, luminance is a function not just of the reflectance of surfaces—that is, the quantity of light reflected by an object—but also a function of both the illumination—the amount of light that hits an object—and the transmittance properties of the space between the object and the observer—for instance, the atmosphere.[43]

For simplicity, we can focus here on reflectance and illumination as the two primary variables that determine luminance. The same luminance can be caused by a dark surface illuminated brightly, and by a less illuminated light surface. Vision has to somehow disambiguate this contingency and figure out what combination of reflectance and illumination is responsible for a given luminance quantity at the retina.

In Natural Scene Statistics, solving this problem means looking at the environmental conditions that give rise to perceived brightness. Consider the effect of figure 2.1. The target circle on the left appears lighter than the target circle on the right despite the fact that the two targets are equi-luminant. In explaining why this is the case, we start by analyzing a large database of natural images like the one depicted in figure 2.2.

We can superimpose the configuration in figure 2.1 on a large number of images to find light patterns (as measured by pixels) in which the luminance of both the surround and the target regions are approximately homogeneous to the elements of the figure.[44] This gives us a sense of what typically causes the configuration that we are interested in. We discover, for example, that, in our world, high-luminance surrounds co-occur more frequently with high-luminance targets than with low-luminance targets. *Vice versa*, low-luminance

43. Howe et al. 2006.

44. Yang and Purves 2004, p. 8746.

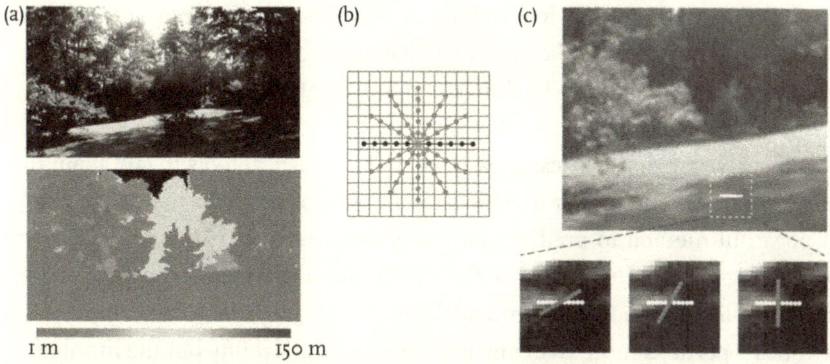

FIGURE 2.2 Example of image of a natural scene. From Purves and Lotto 2005b, p. 28. The image in question was used to sample straight lines rather than brightness patches, but it provides an example of the kinds of images used in NSS.

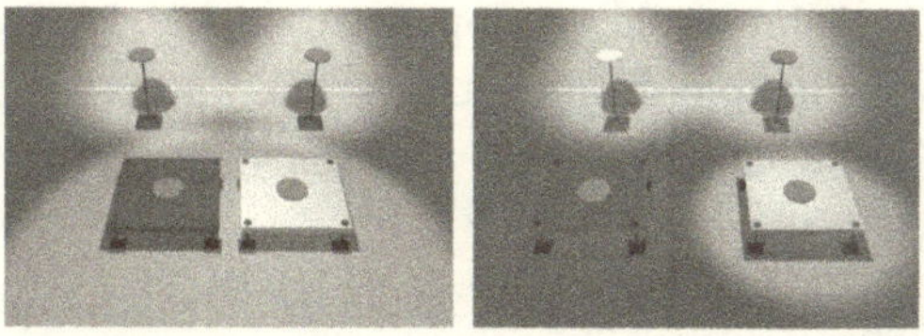

FIGURE 2.3 Two possible sources of the brightness contrast effect. From Purves and Lotto 2011, p. 24. The right scene is, in our environment, the more common cause of the stimulus in figure 2.1.

surrounds co-occur more frequently with low-luminance targets. This gives us a way of interpreting what occurs in figure 2.1.

The luminance of the two center targets in the figure is the same. Given our environment, however, the target that is embedded in a lighter surround should be more luminant. The fact that it is not suggests that it is darker—that is, it suggests that it is illuminated more brightly, and that it reflects less light. Similarly, the target on the left of the figure should be less luminant. The fact that it is not suggests that it is brighter—that is, it suggests that it has more reflectance, but it is illuminated by less light. In other words, the stimuli in figure 2.1 are—given luminance facts in our environment—more likely caused by the scene in the *right* image of figure 2.3. They are more likely caused by targets that are both illuminated differently and that have different reflectance properties. The targets are accordingly seen as differing in brightness.[45]

45. Howe et al. 2006, p. 872. This approach is also able to explain a number of brightness effects including the Cornsweet edge effects and Mach bands (Purves and Lotto 2003, ch. 4, Purves et al. 1999) and we will see it at work in explaining visual illusions in section 4.5.

Again, in accounting for brightness perception we do not appeal to an inference but to the usual causes of a given configuration. If the retinal stimulus is typically produced by things that are different in brightness, then the visual system processes them that way.

What we are doing is, essentially, applying statistical tools to talk about the environmental conditions in which vision occurs. If we do that, we develop a powerful method to predict what observers see. In particular, we discover two things. First, the stimulus for vision, although in principle massively ambiguous, is in our environment likely caused by a restricted number of entities—perhaps more than one in cases of multi-stability but the number is definitely tractable. So the stimulus is much more constraining than we first thought. Second, given the statistical properties of the stimulus, it is unsurprising that vision would become 'attuned' to these conditions—that is, it is unsurprising that vision would develop constraints and biases that make it process information in accord with such statistical properties. So we explain both why people see what they do and why their visual apparatus is biased as it is by appeal to how the world is.

This means that when vision scientists discover the principles that regulate visual processing, they are ultimately discovering environmental contingencies to which vision conforms *via* its biases. The visual system uses constraints developed from past exposure to overcome the inverse problem. These constraints are responses to physical facts that were present in evolutionary history and that are present in the lifespan of the organism—for instance, that high-luminance targets are more likely to occur with high-luminance surrounds, or that edge elements that are co-linear are likely to belong to the same contour. Discovering the constraints, and the environmental facts that shaped them, is the proper subject of vision science aided by the statistical analysis of natural images.

Natural Scene Statistics is thus a recent approach to vision that explicitly supports EV. It is an approach that respects the Gibsonian insight that studying visual perception requires studying the environmental conditions that ground it.

Before we move on to consider another contemporary approach to perceptual processing, and to see how it relates to EV, we should briefly digress to notice that there are different strands within Natural Scene Statistics. We should look, in particular, at a hypothesis called 'empirical ranking theory' because doing so brings out important issues concerning how to understand the goal of vision, and what resources we should use to predict its outputs.

Empirical ranking theory and the aim of vision

An interesting result of NSS, as described previously is that visual illusions, like the brightness illusion in figure 2.1, are to be seen as just what we should expect given the world in which we are situated. The visual system responds to the dots in different ways because, doing so, typically allows it to get things right. Illusions are a sign that the system is wired in the appropriate way given the environment in which it is embedded. In this sense, illusions should not be seen as the product of biological limitations or imperfections. They rather display the (mostly successful) design of vision.

Stressing the 'normalcy' of illusions, some proponents of NSS propose a distinctive hypothesis called 'empirical ranking theory.' This hypothesis highlights the importance of prior exposure and of behavioral success in understanding what we see.

Proponents of empirical ranking theory use statistical methods and the analysis of natural environments to make their predictions, but they reject some substantive claims about perception that other supporters of NSS accept. For one thing, fans of empirical ranking theory tend to more explicitly abandon the language of vision as performing inferences. For another, and more importantly, they attempt to shift the focus from veridicality to behavioral success.

Percepts, according to empirical ranking theory, do not correspond to veridical representations of the physical world generating the stimulus. They rather correspond to what it has been useful to detect in the history of the organism. They reflect the empirical *significance* of the stimulus—that is, the "accumulated experience of what the retinal stimulus in question had typically signified in the history of the species and the individual."[46] We see what we have seen in the past and what it has been *useful* to see in the past, rather than what is out there.

From this consideration, proponents of empirical ranking theory sometimes cryptically remark that percepts are neither correct nor incorrect representations of reality.[47] Percepts are rather elements of behavioral success. In this sense, they claim, illusory percepts are not really illusory, since perception in general is not in the business of getting things right.

Although run together, two distinctive claims can be discerned in the assertions of empirical ranking theory. One claim concerns a presumed lack of

46. Purves and Lotto 2003, p. 10.

47. Purves and Lotto 2003, p. 15.

accuracy conditions in perception. The other claim concerns the fact that vision does not aim at truth. While the first claim is dubious, the second claim deserves further attention.

With respect to the first claim, we should note that the idea that percepts lack accuracy conditions does not follow from the idea that vision does not aim at truth. We may freely accept that what we see is what has been advantageous for us to see in the past, while also retaining the view that percepts can be true or false. The fact that illusions are what we should expect given the history of the visual system does not make them any less illusory.

The second claim, by contrast, raises an interesting issue. This is the issue of how to understand the primary function of vision. The question is whether we should think of visual perception as primarily concerned with *success* rather than with truth. We may pre-theoretically think that the two go together, because representing the world accurately is intuitively beneficial for an organism. A simple version of our usual example illustrates that this need not be the case, however.

Imagine that, contrary to what I have said all along, edges are not the most likely causes of discontinuities in light intensity at the retina. Rather, given only environmental facts, shadows are the most likely causes of such discontinuities. If we think of vision as aimed at truth, we should expect it to track shadows, since doing so would give it the best shot at getting things right. But suppose that, for organisms like us, detecting edges is much more important than detecting shadows. If vision is aimed at behavioral success, then we should conclude that we track edges despite the fact that they are not as likely present. In doing this, we would lose in accuracy but gain in usefulness. Better get things wrong more often if this keeps us safe.

If the example of edges does not bring out this point vividly, we can easily think of more convincing examples involving, say, the utility of detecting predators, or of seeing socially relevant categories such as faces even when they are not the most likely causes of a given retinal excitation. Accuracy, in these cases, may be sacrificed for need.

There may be environmental facts that are tracked and/or represented because they are overall very frequent, but there may also be environmental facts that are perhaps equally as frequent as others, or less frequent than others, that nevertheless get tracked because they are more important for us. It seems that a good theory of visual perception should make room for this result.[48]

---

48. Ruth Millikan (1989) famously remarks that tail splashing by beavers may only very rarely correlate with the presence of predators. Yet such tail splashing means 'predator'

Although this is posed as a problem by proponents of empirical ranking theory, I think that all supporters of NSS have the resources to address this issue. For expository purposes, I used a simplified version of Natural Scene Statistics where percepts are predicted solely by the probability of a given environmental cause, or by its likelihood given what is projected on the retina. This is not mandatory, however. It is open to NSS to issue predictions by using additional tools. Subjects may see what is most useful for them to see. This means that, in predicting percepts, we need to calculate not only what is more likely present given the stimulus—or what is more likely present in the environment overall—but also what is more advantageous to see given some available options. This involves calculating the costs and benefits associated with accepting each percept that has a high probability. Considering costs and benefits includes considering how useful a certain element is for the success of the species. Such calculation may favor a percept with high utility but low probability.

In describing the system as conforming to a cost and benefits analysis we do not presume that the system itself encodes the principles of such analysis.[49] We simply say that, because of evolutionary advantage, the system is biased to process percepts in a way that maximizes utility. In other words, in predicting what observers see, we still ultimately make reference to *external* conditions. We make reference to what is more frequent in the environment, and to what is advantageous or valuable for observers given their needs. We do not commit to the idea that the visual system encodes information about what is more frequent or what is more useful.

If this is right, then more needs to be said to assess the differences between empirical ranking theory and other positions within NSS. The disagreement in question brings out the interesting consideration that what we see likely depends on the intricate interplay between the structure of the world and our needs. What the disagreement does not bring out, however, is the necessity to appeal to a representationally mediated process to explain our perceptual abilities. We see as we do because of how the world is, and because of what is important for us given how it is.

To conclude this section, we can summarize our main line of argument. I described Natural Scene Statistics as an approach that uses the analysis of

---

because its doing so has been advantageous for beavers. Similarly, Mohan Matthen (2005, p. 18) points out that objectivity is an 'instrumental,' not an 'absolute,' value for sensory systems. Objectivity is a goal in so far as it is advantageous. See also Shapiro 1993 for the importance of organismic needs in identifying the task of perceptual systems.

49. Rescorla forthcoming clarifies this point in relation to Bayesian accounts of perception.

natural images to study the environmental conditions in which vision takes place. By so doing, and by taking into account considerations of utility, NSS predicts what perceivers see without appeal to an inferential process. Although the visual system must be attuned to the structure of the world, it does not need to *infer* it from poor evidence.

In the next section, I consider another relatively recent development in vision science and reflect on how it relates to EV.

2.4 Bayesian approaches to vision: neuro centrism without representation

Recent Bayesian accounts of perception retain the terminology of vision as an inferential and constructive process. This suggests commitment to roughly the same claims of more traditional inferentialism. I think that categorizing Bayesian accounts as inferential, however, is problematic. My general impression is that the field of vision science has moved away from 'representation-heavy' and 'inference-heavy' approaches to visual activity. Work on Bayesian models is typically developed in conjunction with work on connectionist and neural nets.[50] Networks that train through back-propagation act as Bayesian systems in their routine attempt to minimize error and, as we saw in section 2.2, reflection on networks of this kind can favor non-representational accounts.

Further, Bayesian models of perceptual activity have characteristics that mark some important differences between the processes that they describe, and inferences. Bayesians do not hold, and do not need to hold, that the structures involved in vision have linguistic or propositional form, and their models often aim to describe dynamic *brain* processes that do not seemingly involve any representations.

For these and other reasons, proponents of Bayesian views disagree concerning the commitments of their position. Some see themselves as simply describing a system that performs like a Bayesian observer; others take their view to commit to representational complexity.[51]

50. Clark 2012, p. 182.

51. See Maloney and Mamassian 2009 for a cursory outline of this debate. Somewhat curiously, Bayesian models would have to posit *more* representational complexity than traditional bottom-up accounts. This is because, as we will see shortly, they posit the need for both prior knowledge *and* knowledge of the likelihood of the environmental causes of retinal stimuli to explain perception—not to mention the fact that Bayesian observers are also thought to conform to decision rules such as utility maximization.

I think that this disagreement suggests that Bayesian outlooks, although somewhat 'neurocentric,' are not straightforwardly representation-centric in the same way in which traditional inferential accounts are. A good portion of the present section makes this point. I propose a deflated interpretation of Bayesian models that I think accords well with the spirit of this paradigm. If what I argue is right, contemporary perceptual psychologists using Bayesian tools hold a view that is more friendly to the embedded approach I introduced in this chapter.

Even if this is not right, however—and Bayesianism is to be interpreted as a cognitive approach in the sense of chapter 1—this will not matter much. At the end of this section, I argue that Bayesians leave an important question unanswered and that this question is best addressed by grounding the Bayesian picture in Natural Scene Statistics. Absent this grounding, Bayesianism fails to be an adequate account of how the inverse problem is solved. Understanding vision in Bayesian terms explains diachronic aspects of perception; it does not explain how the visual system produces visual percepts in the first place. So an embedded approach would be needed anyway to explain how the visual system overcomes the underdetermination problem.

I start the section by explaining what Bayesianism about perception amounts to. In doing so, I use the terms 'Bayesian account' and 'predictive coding account' interchangeably. I then discuss the differences and presumed similarities between Bayesian perceptual inferences and more traditional bottom-up inferences. In judging whether Bayesian accounts are genuinely inferential, the central step is judging whether the machinery they posit is, or needs to be, representational machinery, and I suggest that it does not need to be representational. I conclude this section by arguing for the integration of predictive coding accounts with NSS.

Bayesian perception

Perceptual systems operate in conditions of uncertainty. Bayesian decision theory is a mathematical framework that models precisely decision-making under uncertainty. It is therefore a natural framework for the study of perception.[52] In vision, one important source of uncertainty is the known underdetermination of sensory input. The visual system has to continuously solve the inverse problem.

In traditional cognitive models, the inverse problem is solved by first representing sensory data and then applying implicit assumptions that serve as

52. Rescorla forthcoming.

constraints on how to interpret the data. In Bayesian models, by contrast, vision is said to form hypotheses concerning the distal sources of the data, and to assign prior probability to the hypotheses. The hypothesis with the highest prior probability is checked against the evidence—that is, against the sensory input.[53] The visual system generates a measure of the likelihood of the hypothesis. The likelihood is a quantification of the probability of the hypothesis in question, given the evidence. The likelihood—together with the prior probability—is used to calculate the posterior probability of the hypothesis (by multiplying prior and likelihood). The percept is generally selected as a function of the posterior probability. Roughly, if the likelihood is high and the hypothesis was already plausible the hypothesis is confirmed. If, by contrast, the hypothesis is not very likely given the evidence, then an error signal is generated by the sensory states. This signal has effects on whether the initial hypothesis is selected, and if and how it is changed. As in more traditional inferential models, all of the processing is done subpersonally and automatically. It is not something that the subject of experience is aware of.

Because of how they view sensory states, Bayesian models make use of *predictive coding*—originally a data compression strategy—where information is transmitted by a code that carries information only about unexpected variation. To transmit an image, for example, a signal only encodes variation given by the boundaries of objects in the image. The signal does not also encode regions of the image that are highly predictable given the surrounding region.[54]

As in predictive coding, the sensory states provide feedback if there is error in the hypothesis being tested. In the ideal case in which the hypothesis is already probable and it is also very likely given the evidence, no signal is produced. If there is error, however, the system reallocates probabilities in light of the sensory data and selects, rejects, or adjusts the initial hypothesis as the percept.

In some Bayesian models, the final decision concerning the hypothesis is made in accord with 'expected utility maximization,' which involves calculating the costs and benefits associated with accepting a given hypothesis. In others, it is made simply as a function of the posterior probability of the hypothesis.[55] For simplicity, in what follows, I assume this second option.

---

53. Hohwy et al. 2008, p. 5.

54. Clark 2012, p. 182, Shi and Sun 1999.

55. Maloney and Mamassian 2009, Hohwy et al. 2008, p. 2; Mamassian et al. 2002, p.20–21. The visual system may conform to the 'maximum a posteriori' rule by picking the hypothesis with the highest posterior, or it might conform to 'probability matching,' a non-deterministic

We can illustrate this framework by giving a few more specific examples. Bayesian models have been used to explain a variety of visual processes including retinal responses and color constancy,[56] and they have also been used to describe how human action is generated, but I ignore that literature here. For our purposes, we can focus on some of the more sophisticated visual cases, such as binocular rivalry and shape from shading. In both cases, the stimulus for vision is ambiguous, and the visual system solves the ambiguity by engaging in a process that reduces uncertainty.

Binocular rivalry with predictive coding

Binocular rivalry is a type of multi-stability where percepts shift during prolonged viewing of a figure or object, but it is multi-stability that is induced by the stimulus.[57] In rivalry, the two eyes are exposed to different inputs through an experimental setup that isolates one eye from the other. Observers may be presented with the image of a house in one eye and the image of a face in the other. Subjects are given two incongruent inputs that appear to occupy the same spatio-temporal location. Rather than fusing the two into a single percept—something that sometimes happens, but not for very long periods of time—observers experience a shift between the two.

Bayesian models seemingly explain both the selection of one percept and the alternation between the two quite elegantly. The idea is to view the visual system as engaging in a process of hypothesis formation and confirmation where prior knowledge of the world plays a crucial role. In the example at hand, the central hypotheses in play may be (a) a face is present, (b) a house is present, and (c) both a face and a house are present.

Suppose that, for some reason, the hypothesis that there is a face has a higher initial probability, and so it is the one tested first. If, following Hohwy et al. 2008, we mark the hypothesis that there is a face with F, and the hypothesis that there is a house with H, then the prior probability of F is higher that that of H: $p(F) > p(H)$. Notice also that the prior probability of F is higher

---

rule according to which hypotheses with high posterior probabilities are selected more often than those with lower posterior probabilities (Mamassian and Landy 1998).

56. Brainard 2009, Hosoya et al. 2005. I leave aside the issue of how faithful the models outlined here are to the notions of Bayesian decision theory. Interested readers can refer to the discussion in Mamassian et al. 2002, p. 29.

57. Other kinds of multi-stability—such as the kind that occurs in the presence of figures like the duck-rabbit—are not as 'induced by the stimulus' because subjects are presented with a single image. I discuss this type of multi-stability in section 4.7.

than the probability of there being both a face and a house: $p(F) > p(F+H)$. This is because it is very unlikely, in our environment, to find both a house and a face in the same spatio-temporal location. In fact, it is in general very unlikely to find two or more objects in the same place at the same time, so hypotheses that predict this kind of situation are consistently assigned a low prior probability. This is due to what Bayesians call 'hyperpriors,' or generic assumptions that concern not specific objects—such as faces and houses—but the environmental causes of sensory input more generally.[58]

Going back to the hypothesis F that is being tested. The hypothesis explains a lot of the evidence generated by the stimuli—that is, the images of the face and the house. It does not explain all of the evidence, however, since it does not account for the stimulus that comes from the house. This results in a relatively low likelihood and in a fairly significant error signal. Still, provided that the prior probability of F is high enough, the observer initially experiences a face, and this hypothesis inhibits the competing hypotheses.

Notice that the likelihood of $F+H$ given the input I is higher than the likelihood of the other two individual hypotheses: $p(I/F+H) > p(I/F) = p(I/H)$. This is because the input is much more compatible with the hypothesis that there is both a face and a house than with the hypothesis that only one of those things is present. So the priors and hyperpriors have a big role in making the face win over the other hypotheses.

Despite the fact that the face initially wins, the large error signal for that hypothesis makes a face-only percept particularly unstable and is eventually responsible for the shift to a new percept. A visual system that is continuously looking to minimize error is likely, when the error signal is significant, to try out different hypotheses that accommodate the error. This explains why a different hypothesis is selected and, as a result, why subjects may move from experiencing the face to experiencing the house. A similar picture can be applied to the case of shape from shading to which we turn next.

Shape from shading with predictive coding

Shading is one of the cues that our visual apparatus uses to derive the three-dimensional shape of an object from its two-dimensional retinal projection. Simple dots may look convex because of how they are shaded.[59]

Importantly, however, the configuration in figure 2.4—and the stimulus that it produces—is also compatible with the dots being concave spherical

58. Howhy et al. 2008, p. 5, Mamassian et al. 2002.

59. Ramachandran 1988.

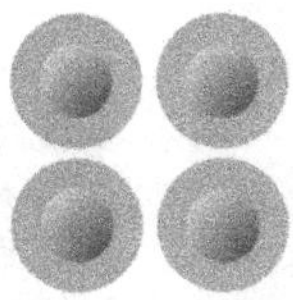

FIGURE 2.4 Shaded dots typically seen as convex.

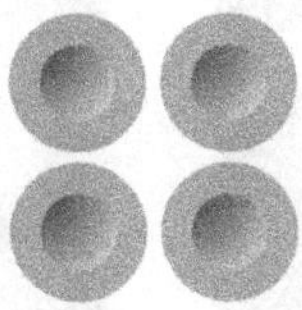

FIGURE 2.5 Shaded dots typically seen as concave.

cavities. In particular, the configuration is compatible with the dots being concave and illuminated from below. What is crucial to how the dots look is not just how they are shaded but how they are illuminated and perceived to be illuminated. If illumination comes from above, the dots look convex. *Vice versa*, if the illumination comes from below, they look concave. This is often illustrated by the fact that, if we keep the illumination fixed—that is, as coming from above—and we rotate the figure, we are more likely to see the dots as concave (see figure 2.5).

So given the configuration in figure 2.4, we could perceive either convex spheres illuminated from above (hypothesis 1) or concave spherical cavities illuminated from below (hypothesis 2). Again, in a Bayesian framework, the visual system *decides* between these two hypotheses.

Assuming that there are no additional cues concerning the direction of light in the figure, the two hypotheses are equally as likely given the evidence. The visual system, however, assigns higher initial probability to the fact that light comes from a single source and from *above*. This is, again, a hyperprior in action, as the visual apparatus assumes a general fact about incoming stimuli, namely, that they are illuminated from a single source above them—for instance, from the sun.[60] So, despite the fact that the likelihood of each of the two hypotheses is the same given the evidence, the posterior probability that the shapes in figure 2.4 are convex is higher than the posterior probability that they are concave. This explains why we see them that way.

---

60. Mamassian et al. 2002, Ramachandran 1988, Rescorla forthcoming, Stone 2011, p. 179. The assumption is actually that light comes from above and *slightly to the left* (Mamassian et al. 2002) but we can ignore this complication for the moment.

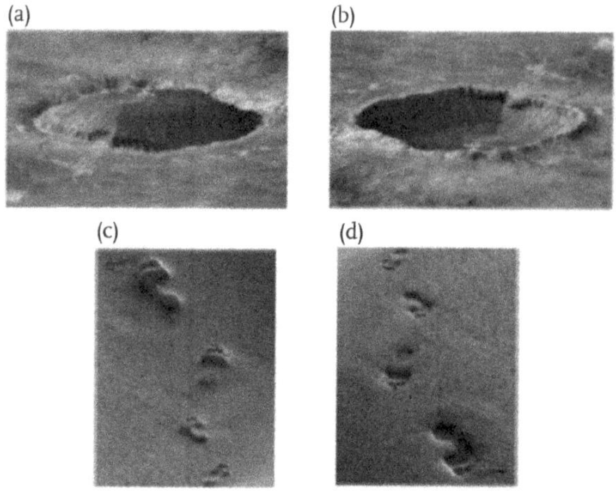

FIGURE 2.6 Natural scene stimuli that appear different depending on where the light is assumed to come from. From Stone and Pascalis 2010, p. 1255.

Similarly, supposing again that there are no cues in the image concerning where light comes from, the rotated dots in figure 2.5 are ambiguous between concave shapes illuminated from above and convex ones illuminated from below. As far as the stimulus goes, both percepts are equally likely. Vision assumes that light comes from above, however. So, the dots are seen, in this case, as spherical concavities.

Natural scenes demonstrate the hyperprior that assigns higher probability to light coming from above even more vividly (see figure 2.6). The same image looks convex or concave depending on its orientation because the visual system presumably encodes the fact that light comes from above.[61]

In the foregoing examples, I gave descriptions of Bayesian accounts in fairly rich terms. I talked of 'hypotheses,' 'evidence,' 'knowledge,' and 'assumptions,' and this may suggest that Bayesian models are committed to the same posits of inferentialism. I want to start looking, however, at three important dissimilarities between these models and their predecessors.

Predictive coding and bottom-up inferences: differences

The first striking difference between traditional and Bayesian inferences is that the metaphor of a 'construction' does not straightforwardly fit Bayesian models.

61. While there is relative agreement that vision uses a prior concerning light coming from above, there is substantial disagreement concerning the prior for convexity. It is not clear that the visual system is prone to prefer convex shapes to concave ones. For discussion, see Stone 2011, p. 179.

The process of selecting a percept is hardly describable as a construction since it does not proceed, like in more traditional models (and like in real construction sites) from the bottom up. It is not a process that moves from sensory stimulation to a hypothesis about the environment in a serial fashion, like when, in building a house, we start from the foundations and then build a floor at a time until we get to the roof. Bayesian inferences are rather top-down processes, where we start with hypotheses concerning the environmental causes of the stimulus and then test them against the evidence.

In the perceptual cases we discussed, vision entertains hypotheses concerning environmental entities, assigns prior probability to them, and then checks the hypotheses against sensory input for confirmation. The hypotheses, in these cases, are representations with fairly rich content, since they stand for distal entities, but it is not clear how these hypotheses are arrived at. They seem to be obtained as simple direct responses to incoming stimuli.

Traditional inferential models tell us how the hypotheses are built out of sensory states, and out of constraints on how to interpret such states. Bayesian accounts, by contrast, only tell us how—and according to what rules—the visual system selects a hypothesis among many *once the hypothesis is there to be entertained.* They do not account for how the high-level states are derived from underdetermined sensation. This is indeed an issue that will become relevant later.

Sensation can play a secondary role in Bayesian models in the following sense. The notion of a prior is crucial to such models, so much so that if the prior probability of a hypothesis is particularly high, that hypothesis may be selected no matter the stimulus because "no amount of sensory data can beat the prior."[62] Percepts, in this picture, are merely selected. They are not constructed from sensory stimulation. So Bayesian accounts are hardly describable as constructive views when compared to their bottom-up predecessors.

The second important difference is that although Bayesian frameworks treat sensory input as if it were data or evidence, such frameworks do not consistently describe early visual states in detecting or representational terms.[63] This is because Bayesianism uncovers an often overlooked function of early visual stimulation: signaling error.

62. Mamassian et al. 2002, p. 22.

63. See Rescorla, forthcoming, p. 25, Clark 2012, pp. 182–183, and Hohwy et al. 2008, p. 688. I say that they do not *consistently* describe the input in representational terms because, in some cases, they do, and we will discuss this issue later in this section. Clark, for example, following Spratling 2008 (p. 8) points out that early visual states serve both an error and a representational function. See Clark, 2012, p. 187.

Sensory stimulation, traditionally understood, has a feature-detector role. It informs about the proximal causes of sensory input. The primary visual cortex is regarded as a site of simple, feature-tracking cells with fixed receptive fields—such as edge cells.

Bayesian accounts of perception, however, suggest that sensory states are primarily error or difference detectors. They inform concerning not (or not only) what is present proximally but also about the 'surprisal' or the discrepancy between their current activation and what is expected given the hypothesis. They have a function *internal* to the system; they do not inform solely concerning what is outside the system. Derivatively, low-level visual states inform the system about whether the hypothesis being tested should be changed or preserved.[64]

We may naturally wonder whether states that signal error are representations. One thing to notice is that the error signal may be quite informative.[65] It presumably does not just encode the amount of error present in the currently considered hypothesis but also informs about what aspects of the hypothesis are wrong.

Understanding error states as representations is not mandatory, however, and it is not suggested by the evidence we currently have. Low-level visual states in a Bayesian system appear to communicate the kind of error present by gradually attempting to reconfigure the hypothesis entertained. Like in an artificial neural network, the process of error reduction is a gradual process of changing and checking, rather than a process where a well-defined error code causes a clear-cut change.

In binocular rivalry, for example, where the error is significant, the shift between percepts is often gradual, and subjects may experience features of both stimuli simultaneously. Elements of both percepts appear together because sensory units are trying to reconfigure and update the high-level hypothesis. At present, we have little evidence for the existence of a separate cluster of neuronal states that independently serve as error signals.[66]

Against this background, it is unsurprising that Bayesian accounts make sense of error reduction in the brain by appeal to the framework of 'free

---

64. Clark 2012, p. 191. In this sense, such states can be seen as concerned with their own, and the brain's, well-being. They inform the brain concerning the need to adjust its own states to reach equilibrium. They are 'narcissistic' detectors in the sense outlined in Akins 1996.

65. Clark 2012, p. 202 n.9.

66. Clark 2012, p. 192, Friston 2005, Summerfield and Egner 2009.

energy minimization.' Free thermodynamic energy is a concept of statistical physics and it stands for the measure of energy 'available to do useful work.'[67] Reducing free energy amounts to reducing the error of the presently winning hypothesis, but such energy is a physical quantity that need not be seen as representing anything.

We will come back later to the question of whether early visual states also have a more traditional representational function—standing for what is external to the system. I argue that they do not since some stages of Bayesian processing can be understood in terms of tracking. The fact that early vision is primarily in the business of signaling error, however, is an important new insight that suggests a departure from the constructivist tradition. It is a feature of the framework that makes Bayesian inferences hardly inferential, since they do not consist in drawing conclusions from premises about the world. The conclusions (hypotheses) are simply adjusted when warning signs are received.[68]

Consider, finally, the third source of difference with bottom-up inferential views: the function that priors and hyperpriors play in Bayesian models. Priors and hyperpriors are often described as a form of prior knowledge held by visual systems and they may be seen as a major source of *similarity* with traditional cognitive views. This, however, is a misunderstanding caused, in part, by the language that Bayesians themselves use. Priors are unlike the implicit assumptions of bottom-up accounts in that they do not serve as *premises* for visual inferences.

Recall that, in Bayesian models, some hypotheses are initially preferred to others because the visual system is skewed to prefer them by *encoding* priors.[69] The language of encoding priors evokes the inferentialist idea of 'encoding knowledge' about the world. As in other inferentialist accounts, priors impact

---

67. Clark 2012, p. 186, Friston 2010, Friston and Stephan 2007.

68. The characterization of early vision as signaling error makes sense of some otherwise surprising evidence. Rao and Sejnowski found that cortical cells respond strongly to an oriented stimulus but do so less strongly when the stimulus is surrounded by other stimuli with matching orientation. *Vice versa*, the response is enhanced when the orientation of the stimulus is orthogonal to that of the surrounding context (Rao and Sejnowski 2002). This suggests that the cells signal error rather than some fixed feature. Their response is weaker when the stimulus is highly predictable given the surround. Similarly, neurons in the LGN—the lateral geniculate nucleus which is part of the visual system standardly understood—can reverse from responding to bright to responding to dark in a short space of time because they act as error rather than feature detectors (Jehee and Ballard 2009).

69. Beierholm et al. 2009; Rescorla forthcoming, p. 6.

the dynamic of the visual system according to their specific *contents*, and "one appeal of the Bayesian approach is that the prior is represented explicitly."[70]

Notice, however, that priors serve a different function than the assumptions in traditional inferential accounts. They are not used as premises in perceptual inferences; that is, they are not independent structures that enter into formal/semantic transitions with the hypotheses entertained by the visual apparatus.[71] They rather have the simple function of marking a hypothesis as more or less probable. Accordingly, we have little *prima facie* reason to suppose that priors come in a form other than as simple constraints.

In Bayesian models, priors do not look like contentful states. They do need to have accuracy conditions to perform their function. They rather look like built-in or evolved functional features of perception that skew visual networks toward certain configurations. They are like valves. In response to the environment, they regulate what neuronal arrangements get to be tested by incoming stimuli. They, of course, can be *seen* as encoding knowledge, but that is because, as we saw, pretty much everything that acts to regiment a system can be seen that way. As in the case of more traditional constraints,

---

70. Brainard 2009, p. 25, Clark 2012, p. 203 n.37. A number of passages in different authors use the same rhetoric. Mamassian et al. write:

> We emphasize the role played by prior knowledge about the environment in the interpretation of images, and describe how this prior knowledge is represented as prior distributions in BDT. For the sake of terminological variety, we will occasionally refer to prior knowledge as "prior beliefs" or "prior constraints", but it is important to note that this prior knowledge is not something the observer need be aware of.
> (Mamassian et al. 2002, p. 13)

Similarly, Beierholm et al. 2009 write:

> (. . .) priors are indeed independent of the stimuli and reflect *a priori* knowledge, and (. . .) priors and likelihoods are represented independently in the nervous system (. . .).
> (Beierholm et al. 2009, p. 7)

And Clark says:

> (. . .) recall that biological systems will be informed by a variety of learnt or innate 'hyperpriors' concerning the general nature of the world. One such hyperprior, as remarked during the discussion of binocular rivalry in section 1.4, might be that there is only one object (one cause of sensory input) in one place, at a given scale, at a given moment. Another, more germane to the present discussion might be that the world is usually in one determinate state or another. To implement this the brain might simply use a form of probabilistic representation in which each distribution has a single peak (meaning that each overall sensory state has a single best explanation).
> (Clark 2012, p. 196)

71. Rescorla forthcoming, p. 10.

we would need additional motivations to view priors as genuine encoded assumptions.

We should indeed clear up a further misunderstanding concerning priors.[72] To say that the visual system encodes them is misguided in two ways. One is that we do not need to suppose that the visual system encodes an assumption. The other is that we do not need to suppose—in a more deflationary spirit—that the visual system has a localizable structure that encodes a number, and this number is attached to an entertained hypotheses. This way of understanding talk of encoding priors may be suggested by the fact that, in a Bayesian model, a symbol that stands for a number—a probability—is assigned to a given symbol in the model.

This would also be too committal, however. The visual apparatus may be accurately and usefully described by a Bayesian model without instantiating structures that stand for the numbers in the model. Such numbers may be encoded within the system, but this is an additional claim—not something that simply falls out of accepting a Bayesian description of perception and of recognizing its success. The numbers that stand for probabilities in the model are used by researchers to describe the system and predict what it does, but they need not themselves be encoded *in* the system. The system may simply be skewed by environmental contingencies to prefer certain hypotheses, such that a Bayesian description of it is accurate.

Similarly, we may give a Bayesian description of a smoke detector that is prone to signal smoke—that is, it is skewed toward that hypothesis—without thinking that the detector encodes a number that stands for the probability of there being smoke. Like smoke detectors, visual systems are simply constrained, naturally rather than artificially, to prefer certain hypotheses to others.

The interpretation of priors as biases seems better compatible with the overall mind-set of the predictive coding project and of its practitioners. The project seems geared at describing what *the brain* is primarily doing—that is, reducing error—and it is not clear that this process, as described so far, requires representational structures.

Further, interpreting priors and hyperpriors as biases accords with a number of remarks that we find in the predictive coding literature. Bayesians sometimes point out that priors are statistical regularities that are 'embedded'

72. Thanks to Eric Winsberg for conversation on this topic.

in visual systems by evolution and development.[73] When explaining what is meant by 'encoding a prior,' proponents of predictive coding models point to simple functional mechanisms of the brain. Priors and likelihoods may simply be given by the values of the weights between neural units.[74]

The already-mentioned hyperprior concerning the presence of one environmental cause in one spatio-temporal location is thought to be mediated in the brain by the mechanism of lateral inhibition.[75] This—recall from section 2.2—is the mechanism whereby neurons belonging to a given layer are able to inhibit each other's activity laterally. This mechanism is presumably responsible for the fact that, in binocular rivalry, we experience only one object at a time, since the dominant hypothesis inhibits the others. But then this means that 'encoding the hyperprior that only one object exists in the same spatio-temporal location' means having developed, under evolutionary pressure, neurons, and clusters of neurons that have the ability to inhibit each other. This is hardly encoding anything at all.

Interestingly, understanding priors as simple constraints can partially answer a question that often arises in discussions of Bayesian accounts—namely, the question of where the priors come from.[76] This question seems interesting and problematic if priors are implicit knowledge held by visual systems, as they would be, if Bayesian models were inferential. In this case, we would need to wonder whether this knowledge is innate or acquired, and in what way it may be acquired if it is. It is notoriously hard to explain how knowledge *of any kind* is learned.[77] If priors consist in physical features of the visual system that perform a certain function, however, then this question becomes analogous to the question of why we developed functional characteristics such as ears and eyes positioned as they are. This question seems more tractable in a biological context.

Now, if this means that visual processing is not really a Bayesian inference because it does not encode priors in any substantive sense, then it only goes to confirm that visual processing is non-inferential after all—not even in the Bayesian sense. It is perhaps a Bayesian process—successfully modeled with Bayesian tools—but it isn't an inference. This is, indeed, the conclusion

73. Brainard 2009, p. 7.

74. Brainard 2009, p. 25.

75. Howhy et al. 2008, p. 691.

76. Rescorla forthcoming, p. 10.

77. Fodor 1998.

I want to reach at the end of this section. In order to do that, there is still some clarifying to do.

Predictive coding and bottom-up inferences: affinities

So far, I argued for three differences between Bayesian models and their inferential predecessors. Bayesian models are hardly constructive, they do not treat early visual states as traditional detectors or representations, and they do not treat priors as premises encoded in vision. Early visual states are primarily error detectors, and priors describe functional features of visual systems. The picture of Bayesian perception that emerges is one where the visual apparatus responds directly to a given contingency with a hypothesis, and then checks if the hypothesis is consistent with sensory states.

It would be too quick to stress these dissimilarities, however. There are also affinities between Bayesian models and more traditional views. Predictive coding accounts are regarded as non-Gibsonian and they sometimes identify Irvin Rock as one of their precursors.[78] In particular, there are two features that suggest a representational interpretation. These features are the likelihoods, and the low and intermediate sensory states that mediate perceptual processes. I think that these features can also be understood non-representationally, but obviously there is room for disagreement on this issue.

It is clear that predictive coding accounts conceive of perception as a complicated process, needing substantial complexity. The central question is again whether this complexity must be of the representational kind. I think that it does not need to be representational. To make this point, we can use analogies with the type of processing that connectionist networks carry out. The idea is that, if we can understand error reduction as something that is done by a network that gradually adjusts the strength and stability of its present state, given its biases and feedback from lower states, we may be in a position to see how Bayesian perception is non-inferential. This position should be regarded as part of an ongoing debate concerning how to classify predictive coding models.[79]

To see if my proposal works consider, first, the likelihood function. This is essentially a measure of the probability of a hypothesis given the evidence. Likelihoods, like priors, can be regarded as pieces of knowledge because they seem to consist of information regarding sensory states. In vision, likelihoods

78. Howe et al. 2008, p. 688.

79. See commentary to Clark 2012.

essentially 'tell' the visual system whether the current sensation is compatible with the hypothesis, and this seems to require some knowledge of the usual causes of the sensation in question.[80]

If the hypothesis is that a face is present, but the sensory states are better compatible with the presence of a house, then the likelihood function will be low. Indeed we can see bottom-up inferential accounts as Bayesian systems that only use likelihoods. If the visual system disregarded priors and simply produced the hypothesis with the maximum likelihood given the stimulus, then it would act like a bottom-up inferential system. It would pick the hypothesis that stands for the most likely environmental cause of sensation.

Like priors, however, likelihoods do not need to be treated as pieces of knowledge. We mentioned previously that they are encoded by the values of the weights between neural units.[81] We can think of them as biases that automatically favor a given representation—that is, a given high-level neural configuration—when a certain retinal arrangement is present.

We can imagine again a connectionist network trained to detect something by being repeatedly exposed to it. Such training causes the network to display characteristic patterns of activation where low-level configurations are associated with high-levels ones and *vice versa*. We can then think of a high-level state as 'checking' the pattern of activation at the lower, sensory level where this ultimately just means that the high-level state activates in a way that is more or less compatible with the lower-level pattern of activation.[82]

Checking for compatibility would be what Bayesians often describe as the high-level hypothesis issuing a 'prediction.'[83] If there is compatibility, the hypothesis is confirmed. If there is no compatibility, then the activity of the sensory units constitutes an error signal. The likelihood function can then be seen as a measure of the affinity between hypothesis-level states and sensation-level states. It is an indication of whether the present hypothesis accords with the sensory states given the associations that have been established in the past. The likelihood function, is not a piece of encoded knowledge.

This way of understanding likelihoods can be applied also if we think of predictive coding in a layered fashion. The higher-level hypothesis 'checks' the

80. Mamassian et al. 2002, p. 17.

81. Brainard 2009, p. 25.

82. Clark 2012, pp. 197–198 alludes to this way of understanding hypothesis-testing.

83. Hohwy et al. 2008.

pattern of activation at the closer, lower level that typically causes the activation of the hypothesis itself. In turn, this lower level pattern 'checks' the pattern at the level below. This happens in stages down to the most peripheral layer—the retinal layer in vision.

Bayesians talk as if each intermediate layer down to the most peripheral one is itself a hypothesis,[84] and this suggests that each layer is a representation. As in more traditional inferences, we have a succession of low and intermediate sensory states that represent external conditions.

I think, however, that it is an open possibility to interpret Bayesian models differently. In such models a 'hypothesis' is not *ipso facto* a state that represents. It is rather a state—for instance, an active cluster of units—that generates a prediction in the form of a level of activation to be checked against the lower units. 'Being a hypothesis' in Bayesian models, simply means 'being a state that generates predictions.' So although any given layer may act as a hypothesis, not every layer needs to act as a representation—that is, as a model of what is in the world.

Put differently, whether a given hypothesis is also a representation depends—at least in part—on whether it is about the distal environmental causes of sensory input. In the perceptual examples used earlier the hypotheses concerned distal environmental entities, such as houses, faces, and convex shapes. We were then inclined to suppose that the hypotheses are also representations. Not every hypothesis in a Bayesian perceptual system is like that, however. Bayesian ideas are used to model processes that involve 'hypotheses' but not representations, such as the activity of retinal ganglion cells in salamanders and rabbits. Retinal cells, under the assumption of spatial and temporal uniformity, form hypotheses and predict the local intensity of each point in an image from the values of the surrounding points in space and time. The cells also check the predictions with the actual intensities.[85] But although retinal ganglion cells may, in the sense above, 'form hypotheses' they plausibly do not represent anything.

Merely being a hypothesis, then, is not sufficient for being a representational state. Intermediate and low levels of vision may act as causal intermediaries in the search for error without thereby representing anything. They can be understood as mere tracking states. The high-level hypotheses by contrast, in addition to generating predictions and serving as error signals for

84. Clark 2012, p. 187, see also Hohwy et al. 2008, pp. 689–690.

85. Hosoya et al. 2005, p. 71.

the layer above them, also purport to model the world. They are guesses of what is in the world.

This interpretation of Bayesian frameworks has the advantage of accommodating the deflationary remarks that one finds when reading the literature on the topic. Hohwy et al. for example, say:

> Terms like 'predictions' and 'hypotheses' sound rather intellectualist when it comes to basic perceptual inference. But at its heart the only processing aim of the system is simply to minimize prediction error or free energy, and indeed, the talk of hypotheses and predictions can be translated into such a less anthropomorphic framework (. . .) This optimization or free-energy minimization can, in principle, be implemented using relatively simple neuronal infrastructures.
>
> (Hohwy et al. 2008, pp. 688–690)

The brain is primarily in the business of reducing error, and while it is easy to overintellectualize this process, it is also possible to deflate it and understand it in non-representational terms.

If this is right, then although usefully described by a Bayesian framework, the visual system need not perform Bayesian inferences in any substantive sense. The system proceeds in rough accord with Bayesian norms and the "transitions among perceptual states approximately conform to norms of Bayesian decision theory,"[86] but this just means that the system acts *as if* it is a Bayesian observer. Indeed the framework seems to be particularly good at modeling brain and visual activity because such activity is inherently statistical and probabilistic, *not* because such activity is inherently representational or inferential. So accepting a Bayesian description does not amount to accepting a constructive view of vision traditionally understood.

The moral of this section is that Bayesian accounts have features that support an embedded interpretation. The machinery they posit can be seen as non-representational, save for the hypotheses that end up being percepts. It is, thus, somewhat misleading to say of the Bayesian approach to vision:

> The science delineates explanatory generalizations dictating how perceptual states *that represent certain environmental properties* induce other perceptual states *that represent certain environmental properties.*
>
> (Rescorla forthcoming, p. 22 [emphasis in the original])

86. Rescorla forthcoming, pp. 8–10.

It is not clear what 'inducing' means in this context, but in Bayesian models of perception there is typically one hypothesis currently being tested and being updated in real time. The states that mediate it need not be representations. The competing hypotheses are lateral accompaniments to it. They may inhibit it, but they don't *induce* it.

Similarly, given this non-representational interpretation of the models, we should not conclude:

> One important and, probably unfashionable thing that this theory tells us about the mind is that perception is indirect (. . .) what we perceive is the brain's best hypothesis, as embodied in a high-level generative model, about the causes in the outer world.
>
> (Hohwy 2007, p. 322)

This is not right for two reasons. One is that, although perception involves the creation of perceptual representations, it is not the representations that we perceive. What we perceive is the world even though when we do so we are in states that represent.[87] The second reason this is not right is that perception is not indirect. The formation of percepts need not be mediated by other representational states. Contrary to appearances, Bayesian models do not fully warrant the 'Helmholtzian' description of perception as inference.[88]

Two points to conclude this exegesis. First, as noted, what I provided here is an interpretation meant as a contribution to an ongoing debate on how to best understand the commitments of predictive coding. Second, even if my interpretation is wrong, Bayesian models need to be integrated with work in Natural Scene Statistics. The visual system might be a Bayesian system, but it is also an embedded system. I conclude this section by outlining a problem for Bayesian accounts and suggesting that such accounts are to be grounded in NSS. The issue I am about to raise is a version of the general worry concerning inferential accounts that I expressed at the end of chapter 1. The worry is that inferential views are not really explanatory, since they leave unanswered the question of how the inverse problem is solved.

A problem for top-down inferences

There is an unclarity, in Bayesian models, concerning how the process of forming and testing hypotheses gets off the ground. In particular, while it

87. Clark 2012, p. 199.

88. Ibid.

is relatively clear how the hypotheses get *tested*, it is not clear how they get *formed*.

In typical presentations of Bayesianism, the models explain visual phenomena such as binocular rivalry and shape from shading, by supposing that the visual system entertains and assigns prior probabilities to a set of hypotheses. This set is typically restricted, and the priors are said to operate over it.[89]

For a nice example, we can recall the case of binocular rivalry. In this case, vision starts out by evaluating three separate hypotheses: that a face is present, that a house is present, and that both a face and a house are present. The visual system engages in the process of confirmation on this set. Notice, however, that the number of possible hypotheses that could be formed and entertained initially is very large. The 'hypothesis space'—that is, the space of all possible hypotheses concerning the environment—is infinite.[90] So it is a question for Bayesian models why some initial hypotheses, out of all the possible ones, are formed and entertained. Why does the visual system, in a given context, considers hypotheses about houses and faces, rather than about, say, cats and dogs?[91]

This question is not so different from the question of why a specific hypothesis, from an already restricted hypothesis set, has a higher initial probability. In answering this question, Bayesians typically appeal to priors. The present question is *seemingly* different, because it is a question about how to restrict the initial pool of hypotheses before the operation of the priors. Nevertheless, answering this question is likely to also provide some indication of why an initial hypothesis from a restricted set is more plausible than others. In both cases, we are essentially just asking why some initial hypotheses enjoy higher probability.

We are, indeed, just asking about a version of the underdetermination problem. Bayesian models have to explain why, and how, the initial set of hypotheses is formed given that the information coming from the world is supposedly underdetermined and presumably un-constraining. The crucial question for such accounts is not the often asked 'Where do the priors come from?' But rather 'Where do the initial hypotheses come from?'

---

89. Mamassian et al. 2002, p. 14; Rescorla forthcoming, p. 5.

90. Rescorla forthcoming, p. 4.

91. The same problem arises if instead of thinking of the visual apparatus as operating over discrete hypotheses, we think of it as operating over probability density functions (Clark 2012, p. 188). Here, again, it is not clear how and why the initial density functions are selected for consideration given that infinitely many others could also be selected.

The option that seems natural for Bayesians is that priors and hyperpriors do the work. Proponents of predictive coding accounts tend to describe priors as only assigning probability to hypotheses that are already in a restricted set. But perhaps this is just a quirk of how they describe the examples, and priors and hyperpriors can also be deployed in selecting what is to be included in the set to begin with. Some hypotheses enjoy higher initial probability because we are skewed to prefer them.

The idea is that, in most situations, we are set up to expect certain things. In an experimental setting, for example, we may expect images of faces more than images of houses. This may be due to prior experience, or it may be an un-learned setting. Perhaps, faces are to be expected more than houses in general, not just in experimental situations. Our visual apparatus may be innately set to always prefer hypotheses about faces.

Appeal to *just* priors and hyperpriors is unsatisfactory, however. It amounts, in my opinion, to not really providing an explanation of why some initial hypotheses are preferred. Notice, first, that hyperpriors are too general to do any substantive work with respect to this problem. Hyperpriors are biases concerning light coming from above, and the possibility of objects occupying the same spatio-temporal location. As such, they are not able to restrict the initial set to hypotheses about particular objects.

Further, by appealing to priors and hyperpriors we are essentially answering the question of how the initial set of hypotheses is restricted by simply stipulating that the visual system already 'knows' what to expect in all circumstances. The system is set to prefer certain hypotheses. This, as far as I can tell, is not a satisfactory explanation. The question for any theory of vision is: how does the visual system *know* what to expect given underdetermined input? To answer that it *just knows* is not illuminating. In other words, to say that priors play a role in picking out what gets to go into the restricted hypothesis space is just to say that some hypotheses, in a given context, have *for us* higher initial probability than others, and this is hardly explanatory. The question is (precisely): why do they?

Notice that this is *not* a question about how we came to be biased as we are. This is a question about why a particular bias is active in a given context. We can agree that we, and our visual *apparati*, are biased in all sorts of ways, preferring light coming from above, faces, and convexity. We can further all agree that we need a story of how we came to be biased as we are. The present question, however, does not concern the ontogenesis of bias. It rather concerns why, of all the possible biases that we have, *some*—and not others—are active in a given context. It seems that, in answering this question, we need to appeal to something *other* than the biases themselves.

This is why the present problem arises for unexperienced and experienced observers alike. We can consider fully mature observers who are biased to prefer all sorts of elements at the expense of others. Yet, even in their case, we need some sense of why, in a given context, they consider *some* hypotheses instead of others.

The general issue is that prior knowledge, expectations, and biases cannot do the work *by themselves*. The process of hypothesis confirmation has to be set in motion somehow, and this requires some hypotheses to start with. The visual system must be triggered to expect *something* and it is hard to make sense of how this triggering happens without appeal to information coming 'from the bottom.' It is plausible to suppose, for example, that when exposed to images of faces, the visual system entertains hypotheses about faces *precisely because* it is exposed to them.

Proponents of Bayesian models sometime remark on the role of the 'driving signal.'[92] Appeal to a driving signal typically occurs in the context of explaining how we are capable of seeing *surprising* things—that is, things that are contrary to what we expect. It seems, however, that such appeal is needed even when what we see is not surprising in any interesting sense of the term. Seeing the image of a house wouldn't be more surprising than seeing the image of a face in an experimental situation.

But, if Bayesians appeal to the 'driving signal,' then their model is in trouble as a single explanatory model of perceptual processing. Notice, first, that the 'driving signal' suggestion is somewhat problematic in Bayesian accounts where the information coming from low-level vision has primarily an error-detector function. In order to drive anything, the signal coming from early vision would have to perform the more traditional function of detecting what is outside the perceiver.

Additionally, it is not clear what this proposal would mean for a Bayesian framework that accepts the fundamental ambiguity of the visual stimulus. If the stimulus is radically underdetermined, then it is ill-suited to produce a signal that could 'drive' a restricted number of percepts. Supposedly, it is precisely because the stimulus is inadequate that we need the Bayesian framework. Predictive coding runs the risk, here, of requiring some kind of bottom-up explanation.

Indeed, if we appeal to the driving signal, then it is unclear why the Bayesian model is needed *at all*. If the initial set of hypotheses is, in many

---

92. Clark 2012, pp. 190, 196–197. Dopamine release is thought to play a role in assigning high reliability to the signal.

contexts, restricted by the signal, then it is the signal that solves most of the underdetermination problem and that plays a central role in establishing which hypotheses are initially more plausible. The subsequent top-down testing of a restricted set is only an accompaniment to this initial process.

It is for this reason that I think that Bayesian accounts of perception need to be grounded in Natural Scene Statistics. Such accounts do not constitute a single solution to the inverse problem. They need to be integrated with some other story of how underdeterminacy is overcome. Appeal to external regularities can do it. The sensory stimulus, although underdetermined in principle, is, in our environment, only compatible with one or a few other causes, as discovered by analyzing natural scenes. This, combined with considerations of utility, explains why the brain is likely to entertain only one or a few hypotheses when exposed to the stimulus. The subsequent testing of a restricted number of hypotheses is a simple accompaniment to this initial selection. Priors do not do work by themselves.[93]

The possibility of combining predictive coding to Natural Scene Statistics is obfuscated by the fact that the two approaches are sometimes described as alternatives.[94] I think that this is a misunderstanding fostered, in part, by the fact that some proponents of NSS openly reject Bayesian models,[95] and by the fact that Bayesianism tends to be overintellectualized and classified as a constructive view. If what I said in this subsection is right, not only are accounts of vision based on NSS compatible with predictive coding accounts, but they constitute a needed addition to them. The two outlooks on how to explain visual processing can go hand in hand and they account for both how the inverse problem is solved and how a stable percept is maintained.

Appeal to external conditions explains why vision prefers one hypothesis over others and achieves initial perceptual stability. The predictive coding insight that the brain is primarily interested in reducing error helps explain

---

93. Strictly speaking, the point I am making is that Bayesian accounts need to be grounded in something else. I argue for grounding them in NSS, because I find this approach plausible, and because it respects what happens in some of vision science (see Geisler 2008). One can argue, however, for integrating predictive coding with other approaches—for example, with an understanding of the relation between perception and action, where action has a role in restricting the initial hypothesis space. I doubt that the resulting view would be able to address the issue I raise without appeal to NSS, but developing this point would take me too far afield. Thanks to Jenny Judge and Casey O'Callaghan for pressing this point.

94. Clark 2012, p. 203 n.23. Nevertheless, Clark (personal communication) agrees that Bayesian predictive coding models require grounding in NSS.

95. Howe et al. 2006.

how stability is retained over time. Such insight helps explain *diachronic* perception. Prolonged viewing may change the way something looks because although what we see is determined by what we are exposed to, and have been exposed to, the visual system continuously adjusts in an attempt to reduce error. This continuous attempt also explains instability when the stimulus for vision is less constraining and ambiguous. This gives us a powerful embedded model of both how visual percepts are produced directly and how they are maintained over time.

2.5 Conclusion

This chapter described in some detail an embedded account of visual processing, according to which visual perception does not employ representational resources to produce visual percepts. Since no representations are employed, vision produces percepts *directly*. It is important to remark, however, that this embedded position does not hold that *no* processing at all is involved in the formation of percepts. It rather holds that such processing does not consist of an inference. Vision can be explained by appeal to functional states and features that are not representations. It is direct in this sense.

I further argued that this way of understanding visual perception is supported by, and compatible with, recent developments in vision science. Bayesian models of perception, although typically described as constructive, have features that favor a less intellectualized interpretation. If we follow, further, the insights of Natural Scene Statistics, we end up understanding the visual system as placed in a highly structured environment that shaped it—and continues to shape it—to function in a certain way. The statistical properties of the stimulus ultimately explain why we see the world as we do.

This chapter served as a first step in establishing the theoretical plausibility of the embedded view. Chapter 3 continues this task by discussing the notion of implicit representation and by expanding on the argument for the distinction between representations and states that merely track. The chapter then starts to analyze the issue of the empirical plausibility of EV by arguing that we do not have evidence for supposing that intermediate visual states are representations. Chapter 4 is devoted to refining this argument by showing that EV has considerable explanatory power. Chapter 5 concludes with a discussion of the notion of computation and the sense in which embedded visual systems are computational systems.

3

Representation and the issue of evidence

Hence, the test is that, by viewing the device as transforming physical patterns of inputs into physical patterns of outputs, we lose no explanatory power, inasmuch as everything that must be accounted for—all relevant generalizations—can be captured in an account that makes no mention of what various properties and states represent.

(ZENON PYLYSHYN 1984, p. 26)

There is nothing more basic to intentionality than this pattern of coming together and coming apart, at one moment being fully engaged, at another point being separated, but separated—this is the point—in such a way as to stay coordinated with what at that moment is distal and beyond effective reach.

(BRIAN CANTWELL-SMITH 1996, p. 206)

3.1 Introduction

Chapter 2 introduced a situated way of understanding visual processing and argued that it accords well with current research on vision in cognitive psychology. The embedded model emerges from understanding visual operations as placed in a structured environment, and from keeping functional states and features of the visual apparatus separate from representational states and features. We should distinguish, in particular, a perceptual bias (or a constraint) from an encoded assumption (or an encoded rule or a represented principle), and a state that tracks from one that represents. Biases and constraints that regulate visual processing, and early visual states that merely respond to the environment, are not properly seen as representations.

This chapter defends these distinctions. The difference between an encoded assumption and a constraint is sometimes obfuscated by the notion of implicit representation. Knowledge, assumptions, and principles are said to be represented only *implicitly* in visual systems. This presumably makes the claim that they are encoded more plausible, and can be taken to suggest that the embedded view is not a genuine empirical hypothesis, as it does not sufficiently differ from a qualified sort of inferentialism. Section 3.2 surveys a number of ways of understanding implicit representation and argues that they all commit inferentialists to what EV says is not needed. To make inferentialism into a distinctive empirical view, implicit representations need to be representations in a robust enough sense, but this comes at the price of supposing that internal features are not just functional elements.

The further claim concerning early visual states not being representations also needs defending. As we saw in section 1.2, although most theorists agree on the basic features of representational states (standing in, informing, and performance-contribution) there is disagreement concerning their additional properties—for instance, whether they are language-like or sign-like structures. We may find it implausible to suppose that vision is mediated by representations in a committal sense—that is, we may think it unlikely that sensory states have linguistic structure. Nevertheless, early visual states seem to qualify perfectly well as deflated representations. They are states that carry information concerning proximal conditions, and they likely evolved to do so. This is arguably true even if we follow predictive coding accounts of perception. If such accounts are correct, early vision serves the double function of signaling error and of informing about the proximal world.

I then need to provide some reasons to suppose that sensory structures are not representations. In order to do so, I offer a more general criticism of deflationary accounts. I argue that deflationary representations are not, in and of themselves, representations at all, and they are better described as trackers. Tracking states are states that are close to their informational origin, and they are typically implicated only in subpersonal transitions. They do not inform organism-level behavior. Thinking that they are representations betrays a misunderstanding of the notion, since representation requires both independence from causal or statistical correlates and performance-contribution. In other words, representation requires, at a minimum, that we *de-couple* the representational state from what causes it to occur or from what merely statistically co-varies with it. Using a Brian Cantwell-Smith inspired (and somewhat poetic) metaphor, we can say that representations are performance-guiding states that do not dance in unison with their causes.[1]

1. Cantwell-Smith 1996, p. 222.

In section 3.5, I present two important ways in which the detachment of representations from their lawful co-variants materializes. One way is when a state guides behavior by standing for something that is not present, in the sense of not impinging on the organism's senses. The other, somewhat neglected sense, is when the state stands for something that is present but more *abstract* than the varying proximal stimulation—for instance, when a state guides behavior by standing for something *distal* and steady despite the flux of stimulation it produces. In both cases, the representation does not dance in unison with what causes it, because it makes moves that the causes themselves don't make, and *vice versa* the causes make moves that the representation does not make.

This proposal, I suggest, respects the function that mental representations are called to perform in the empirical sciences and it reflects an emerging consensus. A number of authors agree that representation requires de-coupleability,[2] and some purported proponents of deflationary accounts, I argue, also agree that a more robust notion is needed.[3]

The remainder of the chapter returns to the question of evidence. The embedded view holds that neurological states and features of early vision that precede percepts should not be seen as representations. Presumably, however—once we get clear on what representations are—there should be empirical evidence to adjudicate this issue. If a structure or state is playing a representational function, this should show up somehow. Those who want to defend cognitivism, in particular, need this evidence, as they are postulating representational resources when the competitor does not.

A problem in this context is that cognitivists and inferentialists often argue in favor of their position by simply pointing to its explanatory power, and/or by remarking that visual systems are describable as inferential. In previous chapters, I suggested that, when it comes to the inverse problem, the explanatory power of inferentialism is only apparent. In chapter 4, I also argue that the embedded view is capable of explaining a number of central visual phenomena. Additionally, I already noted that simply being able to describe the visual system as an inferential system is not a good reason to suppose that it is. Cognitive accounts need additional evidence.

Section 3.6 tackles the question of whether we are justified in believing that some commonly posited sensory states are representations. Section 3.7 asks the same question for p-representations. It discusses whether we have good evidence to suppose that visual systems follow instructions. In both cases, we

2. Clark 1997, Chemero 2009, Grush 1997.

3. Fodor 1987b.

find negative answers. Given some shared criteria for judging that a state is a representation, and that a system follows rules, we come to conclude that vision is plausibly an embedded process.

3.2 Implicit representation

As described in chapter 2, one of the crucial moves of a situated account is denying that the visual system encodes principles or assumptions. Although internal features of the visual apparatus may be seen as encoding knowledge, they are mere *functional* features. They do not meet minimal conditions for representational status, since they act as simple causal mediators. They can be *seen* as representations just because pretty much everything can be seen that way.

Now, an opponent may point out here that knowledge and assumptions are represented within vision only *implicitly*. This is, indeed, how inferentialists often speak. Knowledge of the environmental causes of, say, light discontinuities is represented by visual systems implicitly rather than explicitly.[4]

The distinction between implicitly and explicitly representing an assumption may serve to achieve two related goals. First, it may deflate cognitive claims enough to make them plausible. Second, it may suggest that EV is not a distinctive empirical thesis, since it is not substantially different from its (qualified) competitor.

Despite the fact that there are different ways of understanding this distinction, however, each of these ways commits the cognitivist to more than what EV says is needed to explain perceptual activity. The problem is that inferentialists have to make a claim that is robust enough to retain substance, and this comes at the price of postulating more than what the embedded view does.

One way of understanding the distinction between implicitly and explicitly representing an assumption is to take it to denote a difference between knowledge that is available to the whole cognitive system, including the conscious subject, and knowledge that is not so available.[5] According to this proposal, a principle is represented explicitly if the structure that encodes it is available for use in a variety of contexts, showing up for example, in the subject's belief set.

4. Palmer 1999, Segal 1989.

5. Fodor 1983. See also Evans 1981 for the idea that subjects need not have a conceptual understanding of the tacit knowledge that regulates them.

Vice versa, a principle is represented implicitly if it is encoded in proprietary representations that only function in a restricted domain.

I return to the issue of whether p-representations are available in a variety of contexts shortly, since this is also a test for whether a principle is represented at all (see section 3.7). We should now notice that, although it seems true that the conscious subject does not know (and perhaps would not assent to) the assumptions that the visual system uses to perform its operations, such assumptions have to somehow be encoded within the system.

According to the present proposal for understanding implicit representations, there would have to be an internal structure of the visual apparatus that carries information about visual principles and that serves to inform other parts of the system of what it encodes. This, however, is precisely what EV denies. Biases are mere functional features that do not act as representations. They are evolved features that make a system act in a regimented fashion by causally mediating its processes. In some cases—for instance, in a connectionist architecture—we might not be able to localize a bias. But even when we are able to localize them, we should not see them as features that represent and serve to inform other parts of the system.

A second way to understand the implicit/explicit distinction is to suppose that knowledge is represented implicitly when it is *implied logically* by something that is stored explicitly.[6] Information is stored explicitly when a system displays a physically structured object, a formula or string, or other element that has a semantic interpretation. The semantic interpretation is the information carried by the structure. Whatever is implied by such information is represented *implicitly*. A system that represents explicitly the Euclidian axioms and definitions—by instantiating structures that carry information about them—also represents implicitly all the Euclidian theorems. This is because such theorems are logically implied by the axioms and definitions.

This way of understanding the implicit/explicit distinction is, like the first proposal earlier, not helpful. For one thing, we may wonder whether information represented implicitly in this sense can play a role in carrying out visual functions in a way that would satisfy the inferentialist. Because the principles that regulate the working of the visual system—for instance, the spatial coincidence assumption—would not be instantiated in any structure internal to

6. Dennett 1982, p. 216.

the system, it is not clear how their encoding could enter into an explanation of what the visual system does.

Moreover, unlike the Euclidian axioms and theorems, the rules that presumably regulate visual processing hardly comprise a system where one can be derived from another. The spatial coincidence assumption and, say, shape from shading are not derivable from each other or from a set of axioms. Visual principles are specific to our environment and sometimes quite surprising if considered *a priori*. One of the general assumptions allegedly regulating vision, for example, is that light comes from above and slightly to the left.[7] This principle is discovered by doing empirical tests, not by deriving it from a set of axioms.

Finally, this characterization of implicitly represented assumptions would still mark a difference between EV and inferentialism. For a principle to be represented implicitly in this sense, we would need to concede that other principles that logically imply the principle in question are represented explicitly. In other words, we would need to concede that other principles of which the spatial coincidence assumption is a logical consequence are explicitly represented. This would force us to ascribe more representations than those that EV ascribes.

A third and perhaps more promising way to clarify the implicit/explicit distinction is to say that the assumptions do not need to be stated as logical rules in propositional format. Stephen Palmer says that the assumptions could be "embedded in the pattern of interconnections within a complex neural network."[8]

According to this way of drawing the distinction, representing explicitly amounts to having a formula in a sentence-like form—for instance, in the Language of Thought—that stands for a given principle of inference. Representing implicitly, by contrast, amounts to having the principle encoded in a pattern of connections in a network, rather than in a formula.

This proposal does not help, however. It is true that principles and assumptions do not need to be encoded within a system in linguistically structured representations. They could be stored in map-like or sign-like structures. Nevertheless, this proposal still concedes that they have to be encoded *somehow*. This is what EV denies. EV denies that we need to think of vision as having internal features that represent principles of inference.

---

7. See section 2.4 and Mamassian et al. 2002.

8. Palmer 1999, p. 83.

Additionally, this kind of position appears to misunderstand how neural networks work. As already noted, networks do not work by encoding assumptions or rules in whatever format.[9] The transitions between states of a network are regulated, among other things, by the strength of the connections between the units. We could of course *say* that such connections encode information about the world—indeed, connectionists often talk this way[10]—but this is generally both superfluous and inappropriate. It is not because of the information they allegedly encode that networks behave as they do. The transitions are rather regulated by other features of the connections, namely, their strength.

A sign that this is true is that, if a network fails to do what the programmer wants it to do, it is not possible to fix it by changing a specific instruction. As Paul Smolensky remarks, "failures of the system to meet goal conditions cannot in general be localized in any particular state or state component."[11] This explains why, in programming a network, connectionists are typically not concerned with what a given connection weight represents but rather with how the weight causally affects the processing. Again, ascription of semantic content to connection strengths or clusters is both superfluous and arbitrary, if it is based solely on the consideration that the connection can be seen that way.

Palmer's proposal for distinguishing implicit and explicit representations, then, does not work. Implicit representations are either just representations or they reduce to no representations at all.

There may be other ways (that I currently ignore) of spelling out what 'implicit' means in relation to visual principles. From the current vantage point, however, it seems that inferentialists are bound to admit that knowledge of the world is encoded in some form or other within visual systems. This commits them to a position that is different from the embedded view.

The problem is that inferentialists can try to water down the notion of inference and of representation however much they like, but if they aspire to propose a *substantive* empirical hypothesis, they cannot water it down too much. If visual systems produce states that detect edges in response to light discontinuities, not because of their encoded knowledge but because of some other reason—for instance, because of the wired connections in a neural

9. Ramsey 1997, p. 48. Thanks to Angela Mendelovici for comments on this point.

10. Smolensky 1988b, p. 15, Stich and Nichols 1992, p. 46.

11. Smolensky 1988b, p. 15, cited in Ramsey 1997, p. 49.

network—then the visual system could at best only *be described as* following the assumption of spatial coincidence.

Further, if the transitions that the system undergoes are transitions between mere tracking states—or between tracking states and representations, but the transitions are merely associative—then the visual system could at best only *be described as* performing inferences. This claim softens the inferential position so much to make it fairly uninteresting.

Palmer seems to have in mind precisely this worry when, in a passage following his discussion of implicitly representing assumptions, he says:

> Using the term 'inference' to describe such a process may seem to be somewhat metaphorical and thus to undercut the force of the claim that perception works by unconscious inference. But, as we said at the outset, unconscious inference must be at least somewhat metaphorical, since normal inference is quite clearly slow, laborious, and conscious, whereas perception is fast, easy, and unconscious. The important point for present purposes is that perception relies on processes that can be usefully viewed as inferences that require heuristic assumptions.
>
> (Palmer 1999, p. 83)

Although Palmer moves on to talk of visual processing as inferential, as though he had fully addressed the problem, the passage highlights an important worry for his view, and for any inferential view. In order to be a substantive claim and not a mere metaphor, the inferential account has to hold that mental processes are not just *viewable as* inference but that they *are* inferences. If the claim is simply that visual systems act as if they are performing inferences, then it is a claim that everybody, including proponents of competing ecological accounts, can agree with.

If this is right, then the notion of implicit representation does not threaten the status of EV as a distinctive empirical hypothesis. The embedded view understands internal biases of the visual system as neuro-physiological responses to environmental pressure that perform a certain function, not as representations. It understands the transitions between intermediary visual states as wired, or associative, not as rule-following. It favors explanations that make essential reference to the environmental conditions under which vision occurs, and under which it evolved. We see edges when exposed to discontinuities in light intensity because edges are the typical environmental causes of such discontinuities—and because they are advantageous for us to see. We don't know anything, either implicitly or explicitly, about these environmental contingencies, prior to studying vision. In the next section, I defend the claim that tracking states are also not representations.

3.3 Beyond misrepresentation

The argument proposed in this book depends on the premise that deflationary accounts of mental representation are mistaken. Such accounts fail to properly honor the distinction between states that track, register, respond, or, in other ways, are sensitive to environmental features and states that represent. By so doing, deflationary accounts hold an overly liberal view of what representations are and they fall prey to panrepresentationalism, the position that virtually all systems in the environment are capable of representing it.

Deflationary notions of mental representation comprise both pure informational views, common especially in neuroscience, and slightly more robust notions. These are thought to enrich informational accounts, and they include teleological and asymmetric dependency views.[12]

In this section, I first present pure informational views and their problems. The issue of misrepresentation is commonly thought to be the primary reason to abandon informational accounts. I claim, however, that misrepresentation is only a symptom of a bigger problem. The problem is that of detaching a performance-guiding state from its causal and statistical correlates. I then use this consideration to criticize enriched versions of informational views, arguing that we need to move past misrepresentation to find sufficient conditions for representational status. I end the section with an interpretive point. I try to show that purported proponents of deflationary accounts do not, in fact, hold them. They hold a more robust view.

Information and trivialization

According to pure informational views, a representation is simply a detector—that is, a state that carries information about another state of affairs and causes something else to happen. There are different ways of spelling out what carrying information means.[13] One popular and minimal way is to understand

12. Dretske 1991, Fodor 1990a. Millikan's view is not included among enriched informational views because, in her account—as far as I understand it—information carriage is not a necessary condition for representation (recall tail-splashing by beavers in footnote 48, ch. 2.). The argument in this chapter, however, may apply to Millikan's account of representation insofar as such account is also chargeable with panrepresentationalism.

13. Ramsey 2007, pp. 133–134.

information carriage in terms of causal co-variation.[14] Another way is to understand it in probabilistic terms.[15] According to the first idea, a state *S* carries information about *X* if and only if *X* causes, or would cause, *S* to occur. Groups of neurons that respond to the presence of certain environmental entities are examples of states that carry information in this sense.

Probabilistic notions, by contrast, hold that carrying information may not require causal co-variation. What is needed, instead, is a reduction of uncertainty. A state *S*, in this view, carries information about *X* when the occurrence of *S* reduces uncertainty concerning the presence of *X*, and, correspondingly, increases the probability that *X* is present. Neurons that respond selectively carry information in this sense as well.

Regardless of the specific account of information, the basic idea for this kind of deflationary view is that an internal state is a representation when "the state reliably responds to, is caused by, or in some way nomically depends upon some external condition."[16]

This notion is quite common in some areas of cognitive neuroscience where even individual neurons are said to detect and, consequently, to represent various conditions. O'Reilly and Munakata make this explicit and are worth citing at length:

> The neuron (or a unit in more abstract computational models) provides the basic information-processing mechanisms that are the foundation for all human cognition. (...) The central idea we use to explain what the neuron is doing is that of a detector. As a simplification, we can think of a neuron as detecting the existence of some set of conditions, and responding with a signal that communicates the extent to which those conditions have been met. (...) In the brain, there are neurons in the early stages of the visual system that are constantly sampling the visual input looking for conditions that indicate the presence of very simple visual features such as bars of light at a given position and orientation in the visual scene. Higher up in the visual system, there are neurons that detect different sets of objects. (...) The specialized nature of neural detectors is also important in enabling us to refer to the representation of a given neuron. This term has a somewhat

14. Fodor 1990b, p. 514.

15. Dretske 1981, ch. 1 and 2, Shannon 1948.

16. Ramsey 2007, p. 123.

> controversial history, but it is widely used in a way that is roughly consistent with the idea that a neuron's representation is simply that which it detects. Thus, the neuron that detects an oriented bar at a given position is said to represent an oriented bar at a given position.
>
> (O'Reilly and Munakata 2000, pp. 23–25)

Along similar lines to what O'Reilly and Munakata claim, neurons in the visual system of cats and other animals that become active in the presence of slits of light at different orientations are often regarded as 'edge detectors.'[17] Groups of neurons in the frog's optic nerve that respond best to dark moving objects are considered to be 'bug detectors.'[18] Individual neurons in the inferior temporal region of the macaque brain that fire in response to the visual presentation of faces are considered to be 'face cells.'[19]

There are also examples of this kind of representation that do not involve neural activity. In one example, iron traces found in the propulsion mechanism of anaerobic bacteria are considered representations of oxygen-free water. This is because such traces are reliably pulled in the direction of magnetic North which, as it happens, is also the direction of water that is poor in oxygen. The traces are thus viewed as representations that tell the bacteria where to go.[20]

Although informational views offer a naturalistically acceptable notion of representation, there is widespread consensus that they are inadequate for two main reasons. The first problem is that information carriage is not sufficient to deliver content. This is typically made evident by the fact that information carriage is not capable of accounting for misrepresentation. Representations that are about the world should be capable of misrepresenting what is in the world. If they are not capable of doing so, then they are not representations. The second problem is that, while information is ubiquitous, representation is not.

To see why carrying information is not sufficient to deliver content and to explain misrepresentation, consider, first, the idea that carrying information is grounded in causal co-variation. In this picture, information is tied to

---

17. Hubel and Wiesel 1962, 1968. As Ramsey (2007, p. 120) points out, however, Hubel and Wiesel themselves are cautious about the identification of neurons that respond selectively with representations.

18. Lettvin et al. 1959, p. 1951.

19. Elliffe 1999.

20. Blakemore and Frankel 1981, Ramsey 2007, p. 123.

etiology.[21] If occurrences of a certain state—for instance, a neurological state—have two kinds of etiologies, then there are also two kinds of information that they carry. But then error is ruled out. If certain neurons are caused to be active in the presence of, say, edges but also in the presence of something other than edges, then such neurons do not misrepresent. Since they carry information about both edges and something other than edges, when they fire in the presence of something else, they are correctly representing *that* entity. Accordingly, such neurons could not be labeled 'edge representations.' They do not carry information about edges only.

This is, indeed, a recognized problem in neuroscience.[22] It is well known that neurons respond to a very large number of inputs coming both from the environment and from adjacent neurons. The response profile of the so-called face-cells, for example, is more complicated than at first thought. Such cells appear to selectively respond not only to faces but also to downward movement of the head at a distance and, when the distance diminishes, to downward movement of the eyes alone.[23] The cells are not properly labeled '*face* neurons.'

The variation in receptive field just noted is, in fact, unsurprising if we accept the predictive coding insight that sensory states are partly in the business of signaling error. Sensory neurons fire differentially in different contexts depending on both what is in the world and what the system in which they are embedded predicts. Their firing behavior signals the presence of different things at different times.

If we consider a probabilistic account of information carriage, the problem of accounting for content and misrepresentation does not dissipate. If a state *S* carries information when it reduces uncertainty, and *S* happens to reduce uncertainty about both edges and shadows, then *S*—according to information views—would represent both. In particular, it would not misrepresent edges when reducing uncertainty about shadows.

If this is true, then information carriage is not sufficient to account for content and error, and it is not sufficient as an account of representation. Representations are states with accuracy conditions. In the perceptual case, they are states that stand for some state of the world. When they do so, they should be capable of saying that an entity is present even when they are not caused to occur by the presence of the entity, and even when they do not statistically

---

21. Fodor 1990a, p. 90.

22. Barlow 1995, OReilly and Munakata 2000, p. 24.

23. Perrett et al. 1992.

co-vary with it. In the standard Fodorian example, a token of COW has to mean *cow* even when it is caused to occur by horses on a dark night and/or when it reduces uncertainty about horses on a dark night.

Consider next the ubiquitous nature of causal, nomic, and statistical co-variation, as opposed to representation. On all accounts of information, smoke carries information that there is fire; tree rings carry information about age; the firing pin in a gun carries information about the pulling of the trigger; red spots on someone's face carry information about measles; the distention of an animal's stomach carries information about the amount of food the animal has eaten, and about the amount of gastric acid that is released.[24] While information is ubiquitous representation is not.

This is particularly vivid if we think of the case of mental representation. Representations are traditionally thought to be one of the marks of the mental. The ability to represent is one of the distinctive features of psychological, as opposed to merely physical, physiological, and biological systems.[25]

If we think of representations in purely informational terms, then we end up considering organic systems as psychological or mindful when they are not. And the thought that many organic systems—for example, stomachs—are psychological is not just intuitively implausible. We can explain *all* that they do, not just at the physical or biological levels, but also at the 'task level' of description, without appeal to representations. We can explain digestion by appeal to functional and organic states that are not representations. Supposedly, however, we cannot do this with more complex systems, such as human beings and many other animals. I say 'supposedly' because this is ultimately an empirical question; but it is an empirical question that concerns a distinctive psychological notion.

Reducing representations to mere internal co-variants of environmental parameters means reducing them to intermediaries that are present ubiquitously in nature. While causal or statistical co-variance may be an important component of what makes a state a representation, it is not a sufficient component. Thinking of representations in informational terms commits us to panrepresentationalism, and panrepresentationalism is not just intuitively

24. These examples are in Dretske 1991, p. 66, Fodor 1990b, Grice 1957, Ramsey 2007, p. 136.

25. Brentano [1874] 2009. Representations need not be the *only* mark of the mental. Phenomenology may also be distinctive of psychology. However, I take representation to be what distinguishes *cognitive* mental processes from *non-cognitive* mental processes. Thanks to Brandon Tinklenberg for pressing this point.

implausible. It rather robs us of a scientifically fruitful notion that is distinctive of psychology. It reduces the notion of a representation to the notion of a mere relay switch.[26]

Now, in rejecting informational views of representation, the discussion has centered primarily around the problem of error or misrepresentation. I think that this is because misrepresentation is an early symptom of the possibility of detaching a state from its causal origin as well as from its statistical correlates. If a state misrepresents edges, then that means that the state is capable of standing for them even when it is caused to occur by something else, and even when it reduces uncertainty about things other than edges. What is behind both of the problems we just outlined is that representational states have to be distinguished from their causes and from what merely statistically correlates with them. Representations are not as ubiquitous as causal and statistical co-variations, and in misrepresentation they exhibit their ability to stand for something that did not cause them to occur.

Since information carriage is not sufficient to deliver error, the focus has been on finding further conditions that make room for it. Both asymmetric dependency (Fodor) and teleological views (Dretske) are geared toward explaining how representational states that carry information can also misrepresent. The hope is that whatever story gives us error will also give us genuine content.

According to asymmetric dependency accounts, a state that carries information (in the causal sense) can also misrepresent when there is an asymmetric dependence between the causes of the state. A token of a neurological state represents edges even when it is caused to occur by shadows, because had there not been edge-caused tokens of the state, there would not be shadow-caused tokens. There is a certain asymmetry in what causes a given informational state. Edge-detecting states can be caused by shadows because they are typically caused by edges, not *vice versa*. This is why, when edge-detecting states fire in the presence of shadows, they are misrepresenting the presence of edges.

According to teleological accounts, by contrast, an informational state is capable of misrepresenting when the state has the selected function of carrying the information it carries. Edge-detecting neurons represent edges even when they are caused to fire by shadows, and even when they reduce uncertainty about them, because they were selected for detecting edges. They are

26. Ramsey 2007, p. 126.

supposed to detect edges. Such neurons evolved, and were incorporated into the perceptual system, because of their sensitivity to edges, not because of their sensitivity to something else. When they fire in the presence of shadows they are, in this sense, malfunctioning. Error is a product of such malfunctioning.

There is considerable debate concerning whether either of these views can deliver a satisfactory account of misrepresentation and content. Problems have been raised concerning, first, whether the two views deliver contents that are determinate enough to be useful in psychology, and second, concerning the lack of sufficient conditions for generating veridicality.[27] Teleological views are accused, in particular, of confusing the notion of functioning properly or improperly with the notion of being veridical or 'falsidical.' Failing to function properly is a type of error, but it is not an error that uncontroversially involves falsehood. Many things can malfunction without thereby having accuracy conditions. The firing pin in a gun, for example, can fail to work properly when the trigger is pulled, without thereby representing correctly or incorrectly either the pulling of the trigger or anything else.[28]

I think that these are valuable criticisms that merit serious consideration, but, in what follows, I want to focus on a different way of looking at what goes wrong with asymmetric-dependency and functional views. I want to avoid centering exclusively on the issue of content and veridicality. This is because I think that, even if we grant that asymmetric dependence and function provide *some sense* of how a state can misfire, and perhaps even *some sense* of how a state has content, they do not provide sufficient conditions for representation. Asymmetric dependence and function fail to properly distinguish representations from reliable co-variants that are widely present in nature (what I call 'tracking states'), thus failing to single out a *distinctive* explanatory notion. Even if we concede that tracking states have content in some minimal sense, we should distinguish them from representations.[29]

The focus on misrepresentation has been, in some sense, the wrong focus. It is right in recognizing that representations are performance-guiding states that can occur in the absence of what they represent. The focus is mistaken, however, in thinking that figuring out naturalistically acceptable conditions

27. For the first problem, see Millikan 1989. For the second, see Burge 2010, p. 314 and Ramsey 2007, p. 131.

28. Ramsey 2007 (p. 136) uses this useful example to illustrate this point.

29. Those who think that once there is content there is representation can take my argument to show that reliable co-variants lack genuine content.

for error amounts to figuring out the sufficient conditions for when a state is a representation as well. Rather, I think that accounts of misrepresentation *assume* that a state is a representation and then attempt to explain in virtue of what such a state misrepresents. Such accounts do not provide sufficient conditions for representation. They only explain of the states that we already think are in fact representations, what it is that makes them misfire.[30]

That asymmetric dependence and function are not sufficient to give us representation is confirmed by the fact that they do not avoid panrepresentationalism—namely, the mistake of ascribing representational states to too many entities. As a result, we do not overcome some of the problems that we had with purely informational views.

In both asymmetric dependency and functional views, states that are pretty clearly not representations turn out to be so. This is because many sorts of states that asymmetrically co-vary with something, or that have the function of causally and statistically co-varying with something, have no seeming representational role in a system.[31] We saw a first instance of this trivialization in discussing the difference between rule-following and wired organizations. Viewing a feature—for instance, a direct connection—as a representation simply because it evolved in response to environmental pressure trivializes what it is for a system to follow a rule. It prevents us from drawing a number of useful distinctions—for example, the distinction between associative and inferential processes.

Along similar lines, states that evolved to respond to certain worldly quantities may play no representational function in a system. It is arguable, for example, that the magnetosomes in certain bacteria are representations of oxygen-free water.[32] Even if the magnetosomes guide organism-level performance and can, in some sense, misfire, appeal to representational states seems misplaced. The bacteria merely track and react to what is present. Like in the examples of snakes and ducklings in chapter 2, we can explain what these systems do by appeal to their physiology, their functional organization, and the environment to which they are exposed.

---

30. William Ramsey (2007) puts this point in terms of content. He says: "(. . .) much of the philosophical discussion does not dwell on what it means for a state or structure to serve as a representation, focusing instead on whether an account of content can be provided that is sufficiently naturalistic. I suspect one reason for this is a tendency to assume that an account of content just is an account of representation. However, as we've seen throughout our analysis, a theory of content is only one element of what is needed" (pp. 126–127).

31. Ramsey 2007, p. 131.

32. Burge 2009, p. 314.

Additional examples may help further establish this point. Take the chemical reactions involved in some of our immune system responses.[33] In humans, damage to skin tissue or blood vessels prompts the release of tissue thromboplastin, also called 'tissue factor.' The release of tissue factor is centrally responsible for the initiation of the cascade of reactions that produces clotting. The release is often regarded as an 'SOS signal'—that is, a signal that skin damage has occurred and that the process of coagulation must commence.

Release of tissue factor causally and statistically co-varies with skin damage, and it is supposedly its function to do so. What is more, by administering drugs, we could cause such a release in the absence of damage to the skin, thus initiating clotting through a misdetection of damage. It is dubious, however, that thromboplastin release is a representational state, and that our skin is a representing agent. This is because the release of tissue factor functions as a mere reliable intermediary in the process of clotting. It is perfectly appropriate to view it as just a causal feature of the process. We do not need to regard it as informing the skin of anything. So, even if we can concede that the release carries information, this concession is not sufficient to introduce representations. We can explain coagulation by appeal to purely physiological, chemical, and functional notions—that is, in terms of what kinds of things different components do. This explanation is not an explanation of how skin clotting is *implemented* or *realized*. We might ignore what specific chemical substance plays the role of tissue factor in humans. We might know nothing of thromboplastin. Yet the explanation we provide is an explication of skin-clotting. Skin clotting, as described in commonsense terms, is not explained by appeal to representational notions, and, more generally, it is not the proper subject of psychology.

A similar thing can be said for many other biochemical processes, such as the cellular reactions involved in digestion. The production of gastric acid by parietal cells in the stomach is a response to a variety of stimuli, one of them being the presence of amino acids from food. The amino acids stimulate the so-called G cells to produce gastrin, a hormone that, in turn, stimulates parietal cells.

The production of gastrin could be seen as a signal that food is present and more acid needs to be produced to digest it. After all, the release of gastrin causally and statistically co-varies with the presence of food and, plausibly, it has the function of doing so. It seems, however, that gastrin production is not a representation. It is a state that functions in a very limited domain, and

33. This example is from Ramsey 2007, p. 125.

that simply causes something to happen in a process that is fully explainable without appeal to the notion of representation. Amino acids in the stomach cause G cells to activate and produce gastrin, which in turn causes parietal cells to produce gastric acid. Nothing is lost from this explanation of the process. In particular, the further consideration that G-cells carry information and have content—however justified—plays no role in this explanation.

A similar type of explanation can be given for many other bodily functions, such as vascular constriction, muscle toning, and balancing, where states nomically co-vary with certain conditions. Appealing to the notion of representation, in such cases, is out of place and unnecessary.[34]

As I also mention at other points in this chapter, I think that practicing vision scientists agree that not every neural state that evolved to co-vary with something is a representation. For one thing, representational status typically requires some agent-level behavioral effect.[35] States that are only implicated in subpersonal transitions can be understood non-representationally.

Even in cases in which we have some type of behavioral response, however, vision scientists are not liberal about representational ascription. It is generally agreed, for example, that explaining the mechanisms involved in the reflex responses of the eye do not require appeal to representations. Such mechanisms, however, certainly require appeal to neural states that reliably mediate between the intensity of light present at the retina and muscle reflexes.

In the pupillary reflex, the diameter of the pupil is adjusted in response to changes in light levels, as detected by retinal cells. The cells stimulate neurons in the mid-brain, particularly in the Edinger-Westphal nucleus. Such neural activity is in turn responsible for acting on the sphincter and dilator muscles of the iris. The neurons respond to the amount of light present and cause an adjustment of the pupil.[36] It is plausible to suppose that such neurons evolved to act the way they do, as adjusting pupillary diameter protects photoreceptors at the retina from bright light and damage. The neurons. however, are not identified as representations of light intensity. They merely respond to proximal stimulation and make something else happen.

If this is true, then it seems that both function and asymmetric dependency do not provide adequate conditions for a state's counting as a

34. Burge 2009, p. 316.

35. See section 3.6.

36. The diameter of the aperture can vary between 2 and 8 millimeters. Purves and Lotto 2003, p. 30.

representation. The two notions are in the business of accounting for misrepresentation once we already think that a state is a representation. We should not take them to also give sufficient conditions for representational status. If we do so, they turn out to be, just like their informational predecessors, overly liberal, treating processes that do not employ representations as if they did.

As a matter of exegesis, I think that proponents of what I called deflationary views agree with this position. They recognize that their project is primarily geared at offering naturalistic conditions for error, rather than sufficient conditions for when a state should be considered a representation at all. Accordingly, recent criticism of deflationary accounts as accounts of mental representation are, I think, a bit misguided.[37] The following subsection briefly argues for this point.

Apparent deflationism

In many of the examples used in discussion of misrepresentation by presumed deflationists, we start by assuming that an internal state represents. We then figure out by virtue of what it misfires. For example, we are asked to intuitively accept that a bacteria or a frog represents something, and then we embark in a reflection concerning what makes them go wrong. Similarly, we are asked to wonder what goes wrong when a subject tokens COW in the absence of cows. In all these cases, we start by *presuming* that an agent represents. We do not *conclude* that the agent represents once we figure out what, if anything, engenders error.

I think that this is a telling fact, because it suggests that presumed deflationists are just proponents of naturalistic conditions for misrepresentation. They are open to more robust ideas of what it takes for a state to be a representation at all.

In line with this point, Jerry Fodor recognizes that asymmetric dependence, by itself, is insufficient to avoid pansemanticism.[38] Asymmetric dependence might explain how a performance-guiding state can mean the same thing despite being caused by a variety of factors. Such dependence may ground some type of intentionality, but it does not, according to Fodor, suffice for the ascription of paradigmatic psychological states. Given that representations are paradigms of psychological posits, it would seem to follow that Fodor is not a deflationist.

---

37. Burge 2010.

38. Fodor 1990a, p. 130.

In a line of reasoning analogous to the one offered in the previous subsection, Fodor argues that many systems—such as paramecia and thermostats—have states that asymmetrically carry information.[39] If we take asymmetric dependence to be the only condition on representation, we end up admitting too many things within the purview of psychology. This would amount to trivializing what it is for genuine intentional systems, such as human cognizers, to represent. Indeed, Fodor identifies a type of state that is roughly analogous to what I have been calling a tracking state as opposed to a representation (he calls it a 'detecting' state). He says:

> (. . .) What makes a paramecium a nonintentional system is that even if you are prepared to describe things that affect it as 'stimuli', and even if you are willing to describe the effects of the soi-distant stimuli as 'behavioral responses', and even if you are prepared to describe the causal interaction between stimulus and organism as involving the 'detection' of some property of the former by the latter, still, all that happens when a nonintentional system gets involved in a primal scene is the lawful covariation of a property of the stimulus with a property of the response.
>
> (Fodor 1987b, p. 9)

Systems that merely respond to the environment are not usefully viewed as representing it. This is because, although such systems have states that causally mediate their behavior, the behavior is explainable, according to Fodor, by appeal to the properties of the stimulus to which the systems are exposed. When, by contrast, appeal to stimulus conditions leaves us short of explaining 'behavioral responses,' we are justified in ascribing representational states (more on this in section 3.5).

Something similar can be said of Fred Dretske, although his case is harder to assess. Dretske talks about all sorts of systems—including thermometers and thermostats—as representing, but he also recognizes a distinction between what he calls natural and mental representations.[40] Not all natural representations—that is, not all states that have the natural or selected function of lawfully co-varying with some condition—are also mental representations. Dretske says:

---

39. Fodor 1987b.

40. Dretske 1997, p. 19.

> Not all natural systems of representation are mental. There are, for example, homeostatic and other regulative mechanisms that depend on "sensors" whose biological function is to indicate such things as glucose levels in the blood, temperature in the hypothalamus, and so on. If this is, indeed, the biological function of these sensors, then there are, in the sense defined here, natural representations in the automatic nervous system that are in no way mental.
>
> (Dretske 1997, p. 170 n. 6)

It is rather unclear what Dretske means by a mental representation as opposed to these other kinds of representation. One proposal is that mental representations are only those structures "whose function is to supply information to a cognitive system for calibration and use in the control and regulation of behavior."[41]

Although this proposal is problematic as it appeals to the unexplained notion of a cognitive system—supposedly something that is distinctive precisely for using mental representations—it highlights that Dretske, like Fodor, holds a more restrictive notion of representation. In particular, under this description, states that are encapsulated and do not guide organism-level behavior do not count as representations.

In earlier work, Dretske attempts to capture the distinction between natural and mental representation by appeal to the difference between a meaningful state causing something to happen and a meaningful state causing something to happen *qua* meaningful. Only in the latter case we have genuine mental representation, because only in the latter case we have meanings doing causal work.

Although it is a further question how to single out states that do work *qua* meaningful, Dretske is again displaying commitment to a robust notion of mental representation. In particular, he seems to agree that not all states that have meaning (in some minimal sense) are representations.[42]

If this is true, then alleged proponents of deflationary accounts should be interpreted more charitably. While they are trying to provide sufficient conditions for error, they are not also trying to give sufficient conditions for when a state is a mental representation.

---

41. Dretske 1997, p. 19.

42. Thanks to Todd Ganson for reminding me of this distinction in Dretske. See Dretske 1991, ch. 4 and Ganson et al. 2012.

We can draw a similar conclusion with respect to cognitive psychologists. Cognitive psychologists, like the philosophers we just discussed, are not liberal about representational states, if not in words at least in practice. A long-standing distinction in perceptual psychology is that between sensation and perception.[43] This is sometimes taken to be a difference between what we consciously and unconsciously have access to, or between what we have access to directly and what we have access to only indirectly. The distinction is also usefully viewed, however, as one between states that simply respond to some environmental quantity and states that guide agent-level behavior that is rather more stimulus-independent. What distinguishes representational systems from the rest is precisely the difference between these two kinds of states. In Fodor's words, while we, as psychological agents, have perceptual and representational categories, non-intentional systems—such as paramecia—have, at most, sensory manifolds.[44]

In line with this point, psychologist Stephen Palmer gives a telling example. To explain what is characteristic of perceptual systems, Palmer says that such systems traffic in states that provide knowledge. In so doing, perceptual systems differ from systems that, although optically similar, produce and manipulate only informational states, such as cameras. Palmer says:

> Certain physical similarities between cameras and eyes suggest that perception is analogous to taking a picture (. . .). There are indeed important similarities between eyes and cameras in terms of optical phenomena (. . .) but there are no similarities whatever in terms of perceptual phenomena. Cameras have no perceptual capabilities at all; that is, they do not know anything about the scenes they record. Photographic images merely contain information, whereas sighted people and animals acquire knowledge about their environments. It is this knowledge that enables perceivers to act appropriately in a given situation.
>
> (Palmer 1999, p. 5)

Given the already noted tendency—in Palmer and in cognitive psychology—to identify 'knowing' with 'representing' (see chapter 1, p. 22), Palmer seems to be conceding here that not all informational states of a

43. Goldstein 2013, Mather 2009.

44. Fodor 1987b, p. 21.

system are representations. Not all informational states are structures that provide or constitute 'knowledge.' The internal states of a camera are a case in point. If this is true of cameras, however, then it is not clear why it should not also be true of some of the internal structures of our brains and visual systems. Since such structures merely co-vary with environmental elements, they do not appear to differ at all from the informational states of the camera.

If this is right, then both proponents of inferential accounts of visual perception and those who supposedly hold deflationary views of representation, do in fact accept a distinction between representations and states that merely track the environment. Even if this is wrong, however, and proponents of both inferentialism and deflated notions do not accept this distinction, they *should* accept it. To see a representation as just any state that asymmetrically co-varies with an environmental element, and may have the function of doing so trivializes the notion. It reduces representations to little more than causal mediums. Adopting this position means committing to a type of panrepresentationalism that is better avoided.

We then reached the end of the negative discussion of the notion of representation. I said what representations do not reduce to. We now need to move on to speak of the positive side. Section 3.5 presents a positive proposal. As it should be clear from various aforementioned suggestions, the idea of de-coupling a state from what it causally and statistically co-vary with plays a crucial role in this story. Before we move on to it, however, we should briefly address a worry that seems important but that is also ultimately wrong-headed.

3.4 Is this just terminology?

The last section recommended that we draw a contrast between tracking states and representations. The main reason for this contrast is that representations are not just reliable mediators. We should emphasize now that this distinction is *not* just a terminological distinction. We may call states that asymmetrically co-vary with something in the environment and/or that have the function of doing so whatever we want. We can call them representations if that term is so dear to us. The point is that, if we did that, we would still need a distinction between those kinds of states and the kinds of states that equip their possessors with more sophisticated abilities. We would still need a distinction between the states of our skins and stomachs and the states that appear to regulate the behavior of more intelligent agents. This should be seen as a distinction between functional notions at large and more distinctive representational notions.

These two different types of notions may both be very useful in psychology, even if only one of them is distinctively psychological. Tracking states are not just physiological or neurological states. They are functional states, being defined by the work that they do in a given system. When we give explanations in terms of tracking we are not 'changing levels.' We are not moving from an explanation at the cognitive or, in Marrian terms, 'algorithm' level to the level of implementation. We are still explaining a task described in 'task-level' terms—for instance, digestion or coagulation or vision—but we do so by appeal to functional states that, although implementable in various ways, are not representations.

Similarly, when we explain behavior in terms of tracking we are not switching from explaining behavior to explaining specific movements. We are still dealing with, and predicting, the *types* of movements that bacteria, snakes, and ducklings perform. We abstract from their specific bodily motions. Yet, we make sense of what they do by appeal to functional notions that are not representational notions.

Representations and tracking states may thus be important in accounts of psychological and other competences. The ability to track marks a salient capacity, and it plays a role in subpersonal transitions. This, however, does not make the two notions any less distinct. We can use whatever labels we want to denote them. The important point is to recognize that they are different.[45]

Failing to distinguish tracking from representing has consequences for cognitive science. For one thing, not acknowledging this distinction renders certain types of debates practically unintelligible. Consider the dispute concerning the merits of eliminativism about representation.[46] By citing dynamic and/or connectionist models of mental activity, eliminativists tend to argue that we do not need to appeal to representations in order to explain various kinds of intelligent performance. Eliminativists, however, do not deny that there are states internal to intelligent systems that stand in nomic relations

45. We may, like Dretske, draw a distinction between natural and mental representation (Dretske 1997, p. 170); or, like Rob Wilson, we may call tracking states 'exploitative representations' (Wilson 2004). It strikes me that preserving the representational label, however we qualify it, is misleading, but what is ultimately important is that we keep these two notions separate.

46. Bechtel 1998, Beer 1995, Brooks 1991, Chemero 2009, Churchland 1981, Clark and Toribio 1994, Clark and Grush 1999, Fodor 1987a, Gibson 1979, Ramsey et al. 1991.

to environmental parameters, and that have the function of doing so. They also do not deny that such states cause certain responses. While some eliminativists appeal to the 'syntactic' properties of such states to justify their position,[47] not all of them do.

Anthony Chemero, for example, rightly remarks that one can use a teleological account of representation, like the one of Ruth Millikan, to argue that antirepresentationalism is false *by definition*. This is because any dynamical system can be described in teleological representational terms.[48] Presumably, however, representationalism and eliminativism are competing *empirical* hypotheses. Eliminativsm should not be wrong by definition.

The work of J. J. Gibson serves to illustrate this point nicely. In his eliminativist theory of vision, Gibson recognizes a distinction between what is 'directly perceived' and what is 'picked up.' While properties of light are picked up, according to Gibson, features of the layout of a scene are directly perceived by a whole animal. Although Gibson is not overly explicit concerning what he means by 'picking up,' a plausible way of understanding what he means is that retinal and neurological states respond to properties of light. In so doing, such states 'pick up' those properties for further processing.

Accordingly, Gibson does not deny that optical neurons activate in a lawful manner in the presence of environmental properties and may well have the function of doing so. In fact, no eliminativist denies this. What they rather deny is that such neurons are representations. Failing to see this point amounts to failing to make sense of their position. If, in the deflationary spirit, we take reliable intermediaries to be representations, then *nobody* is an eliminativist.[49]

Further, failing to see a difference between representations and structures that merely resonate has consequences for the practice of cognitive science. In doing research, viewing certain states as representations means asking certain questions about them and devoting time and energy to answering those questions. If a neural pattern is seen as representing, then the focus will be on the kind of information it carries, the kind of correlates that it has, and the relations that it reproduces. Researchers will look for the sorts of other

---

47. Stich 1983.

48. Chemero 2009, ch. 4.

49. Rowlands makes this same point about Gibson. See Rowlands 1999, pp. 108–109.

systems that it informs, the type of storage that is needed for it, and the kind of error that occurs when it misrepresents.[50]

If, instead, the state is seen as a simple reliable intermediary, then the focus will be on other features of the state: its temporal and dynamical evolution, its physiological make-up, and its effects on nearby neurons and on the brain more generally. What sets of questions to ask depends on how we think of a certain structure.

This is particularly evident in cases where the notion of representation gets in the way of good explanation. Freeman and Skarda's account of the human olfactory system[51] and Beer's theory of ants' behavior[52] are two examples of this kind of case. In both examples, researchers found that thinking of internal states as representations was detrimental. Focusing, instead, on the dynamical features of the internal states proved more fruitful.

To avoid confusion, then, it is wise to pick different names for states and structures that simply play a different role. Tracking states are states that are closer to their informational origin. They are states that serve like relay switches. They have the function of causing something to happen when certain conditions obtain. Representational states, by contrast, have greater independence from what they causally or statistically co-vary with. The performance that they cause is also stimulus-independent. What this means is explained in some detail in the next section.[53]

3.5 Representation

So far, I have been arguing for the negative point that representations are not just states that mediate behavior by reacting selectively to some environmental condition. Acknowledging this point is sufficient to doubt that early visual states are representations, since they behave like simple intermediaries.

In order to fully appreciate this point, however, it would also be good to give some positive idea of when it is fruitful to suppose that an internal structure has representational status. If causal co-variation and function are not sufficient, then what is? And why do early visual states not qualify?

---

50. This point has been made by both Freeman and Skarda 1990, and Ramsey 2007, pp. 147–148.

51. Freeman and Skarda 1990.

52. Beer 1995.

53. See Pylyshyn 1984, p. 12, and Sabo unpublished for the stress on stimulus-independent behavior.

In this section, I attempt to answer these questions by presenting a proposal for what representations are. This proposal does not comprise a set of necessary and sufficient conditions, and it is less refined than what I would like. I consider it a starting point rather than a complete account. The proposal tries to capture what is unique of representations by focusing on their distinctive features and on the characteristic abilities that come with them. It should shed some light on why later stages of vision qualify as representations while earlier stages do not.

To start understanding what representations are, it is useful to reflect on the function that representations play in explanation. There is a certain tension in the role that representations perform. It is a tension between the need to respond to what is in the world and the need to guide agent-level behavior somewhat independently of what is in the world. In the typical case, representations are put to work when appeal to environmental variables fails, so it is written in their job description that they should be somewhat independent of environmental causes. If they weren't, they would not be needed.[54]

The need to view representations as somewhat autonomous from what causes them to occur gives us a way of looking back at why misrepresentation, understood in deflationary terms, is not sufficient to individuate representational states. As section 3.3 suggests, function and asymmetric dependence do not provide sufficient conditions for representation and they have trivializing effects. A way to see why this is the case, is to appreciate that states that asymmetrically co-vary with something and/or have the function of doing so are still *too close* to what they causally and statistically correlate with. In particular, the states—for instance, the internal states of stomachs that produce gastrin—are linked to what causes them to occur, functioning as mere resonators. The fact that they can—in principle or just sometimes—occur in the absence of their typical causes does not provide enough *distance* from their antecedents. This distance is one of the central ingredients of representations.

A number of contemporary authors try to capture the distance or independence of representations from their co-variants by appeal to the notion of

54. This way of looking at representations explains, among other things, why behaviorism was ultimately an inadequate psychological theory. Appeal to stimulus conditions was insufficient to explain many sorts of stimulus-independent behavior. Some performance is not a direct function of what impinges on the senses (Pylyshyn 1984, pp. 10–15).

de-coupleability.[55] De-coupleability concerns the need to detach representations from their *causal* co-variants.[56]

A state is de-coupleable, at a minimum, when the state does not require constant causal contact with what it is about.[57] This is generally spelled out in terms of *absence*. De-coupleable states are states that stand for something that is not *continuously* present to the organism—that is, not, at all times, impinging on the organism's senses. It is in cases of this kind that we need to think of an organism as behaving by having something in mind, rather than as just reacting to environmental contingencies.

In what follows, I start by looking at the notion of absence as characteristic of de-coupleability and of representation. I then suggest that there is another notion that is somewhat neglected in the literature, but that is equally as important. This is the notion of a *distal* entity or property. Both of these notions seem to capture what is distinctive of representational structures. Together, they give a good sense of what de-coupleability amounts to.

Absence

In a classic work of psychological theorizing, William James discusses, among many other things, what he takes to be one of the distinctive boundary lines of the mental.[58] Although James admits that such boundary is vague, his basic proposal is that mental life can be said to intervene between impressions and responses when an organism behaves by having an end in mind that is not present to its sense organs.

James provides a number of useful examples. Iron fillings are attracted to a magnet and will move toward it if the magnet is present and if there is no intervening object blocking them—such as a card covering the magnet. We can of course describe the fillings in intentional terms as desiring to stick to

55. See, among others, Cantwell-Smith 1996, Chemero 2009, and Clark 1997, p. 144. In Clark the claim is weaker than the one I am making. A representation is a state that *can* be de-coupled by its causal origin. I argue below that actual rather than potential de-coupleability is required.

56. I somewhat neglect statistical co-variants that do not require causal interaction with their correlates. As argued in section 3.3 statistical co-variance is also not sufficient for representational status, and the points about absence that I make below also apply to statistical correlates. A representation that stands for something absent is a representation in virtue of this very fact. It may also statistically co-vary with what is absent, but it is not in virtue of the co-variance alone that the state represents.

57. Chemero 2009, pp. 48–49.

58. James 1890[1983], vol. 1, ch. 1.

the magnet. This intentional characterization, however, is inadequate because the fillings only behave as they do when they are pulled by the presence of the magnet. They do not try to reach the magnet in its absence—for example, by passing around the sides of the interposed card to reach the object of their desire.[59]

Similarly, bubbles in water rise to the surface to mingle with air. We could certainly describe them as wanting to recombine with the atmosphere, but this characterization is out of place. If we put a jar in the water, the bubbles would remain lodged beneath its bottom without thinking of swimming back down toward the rim, and then back up again toward the object of their desire. The behavior of the bubbles is fully explicable without appeal to an intentional characterization.

By contrast, when we consider mindful organisms, we find that they adjust their behavior given an end that they have in mind, even when the end is not present. Romeo pursues Juliet even when a wall is put between them. A frog in the position of the bubbles finds a path to get to the air—the end it has in mind—even when trapped in a jar. In more sophisticated instances, mindful agents may use internal states that stand for what does not exist at all—for example, children may be moved to look for Santa Claus.

The examples just described are all examples of strong de-coupleability, where the referent of the representation is not present to the senses for long stretches of time, or at all. The referent may be non-existent, or just spatio-temporally distant from the representing subject. In these cases, it is clear that the referent is not the environmental cause of the tokening of the representation. The state that represents is *very* distant from its 'usual' causes.[60] There are, however, instances of weaker, or minimal de-coupleability.

Brian Cantwell-Smith describes the case of a rabbit keeping an eye on a coyote. While the coyote remains in view, the rabbit's tracking system can rely on causal or 'effective' coupling to respond to it.[61] In this case, there is constant interaction between the coyote and the rabbit's perceptual system, and from there to the muscles controlling what the rabbit does. However, if the coyote goes beyond a rock, effective coupling is broken and the rabbit has to deal

59. Since bacteria with magnetosomes work by using similar principles, namely, that magnets are attracted to iron, we may conclude that bacteria are not intentional systems. They are just pulled by the presence of a source.

60. I put 'usual' in quotes because I presume, perhaps wrongly, that, in some sense, Juliet is the usual cause of a tokening of JULIET by Romeo.

61. Cantwell-Smith 1996, p. 202.

with a temporary type of absence. The origins of intentionality, according to Cantwell-Smith, are to be found, at a minimum, in this interruption. They are found when something can coordinate with, and track, something that is not effectively coupled with them. In Cantwell-Smith's terminology, intentionality arises when a behavior-guiding state tracks what is beyond 'effective reach.'

Along the same lines, a frog can track a fly through close coupling. If the causal loop between them is broken, and the frog is still capable of coordinating with the fly, then we can start thinking of the frog in intentional terms.[62]

A similar idea can be found in other contemporary attempts to situate the "fuzzy *but important* boundary between genuine cognizers and other adaptive systems."[63] In some situations, the ambient environmental information is insufficient to enable smooth and successful performance. This is where introducing representations becomes useful.[64]

A telling example is given by skilled reaching. Success in reaching a target object depends upon the brain receiving and responding to a stream of proprioceptive information concerning the orientation, position, and trajectory of one's arm and hand. The problem is that, for fast movements, the proprioceptive feedback coming from nerve endings in arms and hands is too slow. Yet we seem capable of reaching objects, generally successfully, even when the movement is fast.

One plausible hypothesis for how this is achieved is that a neural circuitry is devoted to emulating the real arm-hand system, and to provide mock feedback in place of the absent real-world response. The idea is that there is a neural network whose interconnected units model our arm-hand apparatus. The network replicates the interplay between arm-hand parameters, such as shoulder and elbow angle and elbow's angular velocity. By so doing, the emulator issues the proprioceptive feedback needed for fast reaching even when the body is not yet in the position emulated.

In this case, it is useful to view the emulator as a representation of the bodily system for which it stands, because the circuit acts as a counterfactual presentation. It is a counterfactual presentation that guides behavior that would otherwise be hard to explain.[65] The circuit is a model for something

62. Cantwell-Smith 1996, p. 220.

63. Clark and Grush 1999, p. 8.

64. Clark and Toribio 1994, p. 402.

65. Grush 1997, p. 5.

absent—namely, the projected position of the hand-arm system—and it guides performance by allowing subjects to act on the model rather than on the real world.

From these examples, we see the emergence of the idea that representations are introduced in the practice of cognitive science when a system has structures that stand for absent things. There are, of course, different ways in which an object can be absent. Something can be absent altogether from one's surroundings, or it can be present but hidden, or it can be present but hidden at a given time, or it can be present but partly occluded, or it can be in full view but parts of it are not visible. The minimal necessary condition for an object to be absent in the relevant sense is that it does not, in its entirety, impinge on the senses, and, for this reason, it does not provide feedback—or it provides only partial feedback. Absence delivers instances of de-coupleability, because what does not impinge on the senses is not causally responsible for a state's tokening.[66]

In the emulator case, the body is obviously present to the senses, but its projected position is not, and this is what makes Grush's example a very minimal case of representation. It demonstrates how representations may arise in cognitive structures that do not act as simple resonators. In this minimal sense, something can be present—in a room, in the vicinity, inside one's body—while also being absent, in the sense that it is not impinging, or it is only partially impinging on the sensory apparatus.

This makes the notion of absence a graded notion. Some things are more absent than others. My own brain, for example, is absent in some sense. It does not reflect light that hits the eye, and it does not impinge on any other sensory organ. Proprioception is presumably perception of one's bodily parts, not of one's brain. However, my brain is (luckily) present in a more mundane sense.[67]

Similarly, an object can be in full view though parts of it are hidden—for example, the back of the object. This describes what I think is the normal perceptual condition. Three-dimensional objects are often occluded, but even when they are in full view only parts of them impinge on the senses. We are

66. Unless there is causation at a distance, but I leave this possibility aside. There is also a further complication given by the fact that something can be in full view, and impinging on the senses, while not being attended. I am not sure whether this would constitute a case of absence. It might be a borderline case, but, in what follows, I leave it aside and work with the idea that something is absent if it does not impinge on the senses.

67. Thanks to Susanna Siegel for pressing this point.

never exposed to them in their entirety. In this sense, they are also absent. Insofar as we see them as whole—in completion—we *represent* them to be whole. Completion is an important mark of the emergence of representational states. It indicates that perception allows us to track what is in the world even when what is in the world is, in some sense, not present.

Anthony Chemero has recently argued that cases of absence like the one displayed in Grush's emulator are too similar to cases of mere tracking to serve in drawing a useful distinction between representational and other types of states. Chemero also argues that cases of more radical absence (e.g., the way Juliet might be absent to Romeo) require abilities that are too complex. Appealing to these sorts of cases would restrict the notion of representation too much.[68] So, according to Chemero, we have, on the one hand, something that looks too much like a tracker, and, on the other, something that is too sophisticated to characterize representational states.

While I think that Chemero raises an interesting problem for the minimal cases of de-coupling discussed by Clark and Grush, I am not particularly troubled by the idea of having a restrictive notion of representation. Representational capacities are presumably enjoyed only by a small subset of nature and there is likely a gradual transition from simple to sophisticated representational systems. The capacity to represent may emerge gradually in biological creatures, starting from states that are representational in a minimal sense—for instance, states that stand for something that is present, but not present in its entirety—and then moving on to more complex architectures. Not all animals may be able to think of *very* absent things, such as God, or of the weather in Hawaii while I am writing in Houston. Most animals, however, may be able to represent complete objects when exposed to their fragments, or to represent the projected position of their own bodies.

As for the minimal cases of de-coupling, I think that Chemero has a point, but the way to react to it is not to dismiss the attempt to draw a distinction between tracking and representing in terms of absence. The problem with minimal cases of de-coupling is that potential and temporary de-coupling are too vague, and not strong enough to mark a useful distinction. A behavior-guiding state does not become a representation when it *can* stand for something absent, or when it does, but only for a short period of time. Rather, a behavior-guiding state is a representation when it is actually and continuously detached from its causal origin.

68. Chemero 2009 pp. 60–64.

To start seeing why this is the case, recall the case of misrepresentation. The mere fact that a state is capable of occurring when something other than its typical cause causes it, is not sufficient for representational status. Many states of our immune and digestive systems have this capacity while not being representations. Similarly, in the pupillary reflex, the neurons that control the muscles of the iris could be stimulated by something other than light. If this happened, then such neurons would guide the pupillary reflex through a misdetection of light. Yet this ability to 'mistrack' does not confer representational status on the neurons. Potential and temporary de-coupling does not appropriately distinguish tracking from representing.

A token of COW is a representation of cows not because it *can* be caused by something other than cows but because it *is*. A neural configuration that represents the projected position of one's body is a representation because it *is* tokened in response to something other than the body being in *that* position. The rabbit represents the coyote because its internal state is not caused to occur by the coyote. What makes these cases instances of representation is not simply that they *can* be caused by other elements, but that they *are*. In normal condition, there is a difference between what causes these representations to occur and what they are about. Put differently, even when they are tokened in the presence of what they stand for, representations are about something absent.

The opposite impression arises because, in giving the examples, we tend to choose clear cases of absence (e.g., when the coyote is beyond a rock). The crucial point, however, is that a three-dimensional object can be absent even when it is in view. A whole coyote is absent even when it is not beyond a rock. Only its surface is present to the senses, yet the rabbit behaves as if there is a whole, independent, threatening, moving thing that is to be avoided. In this sense, the rabbit is in a state that stands for something absent. The rabbit does not react to the *facade* of a coyote—what is, strictly speaking, visible—but to a whole moving agent.

Similarly, when we token COW in the presence of cows, the property of being a cow is present. That property is not, however, what affects our senses. The senses are only capable of picking up on things like electromagnetic radiation, pressure in the air, and particles. When we look at cows and token COW we are hit by light reflected by a portion of the cow. That we behave as if there is a whole cow marks the emergence of a representational ability. This is not just because COW can be caused by non-cow things but also because cow-caused COW tokens are not, strictly speaking, caused by cows. I think that this is the genuine—and minimal—*distance* of representational states from their causes.

When we speak of absence and de-coupleability, we should not have in mind a sort of temporary, potential sort of de-coupleability. We should rather have in mind a persisting feature of representational states that distinguishes them from tracking states. Representational capacities surface when a performance-guiding state stands for what is not present to the senses, in the specific sense of not impinging—or not being capable of impinging—on them. We can put this in terms of objects or in terms of properties. Indeed, the idea that some properties are not capable of affecting the senses points to another condition on representational status. This condition is somewhat neglected in the literature, and it consists of the idea of representations standing for 'distal' entities and properties. We are now in a better place to turn to this idea.

Distalness

To get a first sense of what 'distal' means, we can look at a suggestion from an alleged champion of deflationism: Jerry Fodor. As we saw in section 3.3, given his account of misrepresentation, Fodor is concerned with pansemanticism or panrepresentationalism. According to Fodor, ending up with too many entities within the purview of psychology would amount to a *reductio* of any account of representation.[69] In order to avoid this problem, Fodor draws a distinction between states that respond to properties that appear in laws, on the one hand, and states that respond to what he calls 'non-nomic' properties. Fodor says:

> We are frequently implicated in primal scenes in which the behaviorally efficacious stimulus property (...) is nonnomic. Or, as I shall sometimes put the point to achieve terminological heterogeneity: the difference between paramecia and us is that we can 'respond selectively' to nonnomic stimulus properties and they can't.
>
> (Fodor 1987b, p. 11)

Paramecia and thermostats respond to properties such as temperature and light intensity that, according to Fodor, are prime candidates for nomicness. This is because temperature and light intensity are standard examples

69. Fodor 1990a.

of properties that appear in laws—in particular, the laws of thermodynamics and optics.

By contrast, our behavior is often guided by responding to properties that are not quite as 'lawful'—for example the property of 'being a house' or the property of 'being a crumpled shirt.' There may be some laws that we have yet to discover about houses and crumpled shirts, but there are no known laws of the physical sciences about them as such. Houses and crumpled shirts are not categories of physics. They derive their causal powers from the physical properties that they have, such as mass. It is *these* properties that appear in the laws of the physical sciences, not being a shirt or being a house *per se*. A system that responds to crumpled shirts and houses is, according to Fodor, a system that responds to non-nomic properties.

This choice of labels by Fodor is a bit unfortunate, because what properties end up being non-nomic depends on what laws there are. Moreover, what laws there are depends, on the one hand, on what one means by a law and, on the other, on how things turn out. Consequently, whether being a house or being a crumpled shirt is non-nomic is an unsettled question. Those who believe that the laws of physics are the only laws we are going to get are inclined to regard 'being a house' as Fodor does. But then chemical properties would also count as non-nomic, since supposedly there would not be any laws of chemistry. This would make systems that respond to chemical properties count as psychological systems in Fodor's categorization, exposing us again to the threat of pansemanticism.

This suggests that we should refrain from using non-nomic-ness as a label for what cognitive systems respond to, while also preserving Fodor's idea that what is distinctive of such systems is that they respond to properties that seem more 'abstract,' or 'macro,' than the paradigmatic stock of physical and chemical properties.

In perceptual theory, we find a distinction that may be put to use in this context. This is the distinction between proximal and distal properties.[70] The former are properties picked up by transducers, such as the retina, which responds primarily to light intensity. Proximal properties are properties of the stimulus that tend to change continuously as viewing conditions change. Light intensity is a paradigmatic example of a proximal property. It is a property that tends to figure in the laws of the physical sciences, and it is a property that is in continuous flux when it hits the sensory organs.

70. Palmer 1999, p. 313.

Distal properties, by contrast, are those of macro entities and events in the environment that remain constant despite variations in viewing conditions. The properties of light hitting the retina vary continuously, given the state of illumination and the point of view that the perceiver assumes relative to the object of perception. The behavioral response, however, does not vary constantly. We behave as if there is a crumpled shirt—the same crumpled shirt—even if the light that reflects off of it is likely to vary a great deal.[71] The behavioral response depends on the ability to pick up on distal, relatively constant properties.

Such properties do not figure in our stock of physical laws. Indeed, a particularly interesting feature of distal properties is that they are multiply realizable by physico-chemical structures. Being a house and being a shirt are just two examples: being red, being three-dimensional, and being cube-shaped are also examples of these kinds of properties. There are many physical realizations of a cube. Cubes can be made of very different colors and materials, and they can come in many sizes. Systems and states that respond to properties of this kind are different from transducers that only react to proximal and changing quantities.

The fact that distal properties are multiply realizable by physico-chemical structures is interesting, because it is generally conceded that multiple realizability is one of the reasons to believe in the independence and non-reducibility of psychology to the other natural sciences. Multiple realizability is not just about mental states and processes being multiply realized at the neuronal level. It is also about behaviors being multiply realized by types of movement. It is about behaviors being explained by appeal to properties that are not describable in the vocabulary of physics.[72] Mere movements may be captured as reactions to quantities described in physico-chemical terms. Psychology, however, is concerned with explaining behavior that does not reduce to the moving of limbs. Such behavior seems to be, in many cases, a response to multiply realizable, distal properties. It is often a response to what the individual takes to be constant despite the continuously changing proximal conditions.

My proposal is that this *taking* constitutes an early representational capacity. It is a capacity that involves an abstraction. Achieving stability and constancy in perception are ways in which this abstraction takes place. The

71. Fodor 1986, p. 19.

72. Dennett 1987, ch. 2, Fodor 1987a, Pylyshyn 1984.

behavior-guiding states that stand for constant and stable properties are plausibly representations.

Appeal to a sort of abstraction to characterize representational states is not altogether new. It can be found in authors that do not agree on much else. We already saw it in Fodor's proposal that representations are about non-nomic properties. Similarly, Brian Cantwell-Smith, in identifying the distinctive features of what he calls 'registration,' points not just to absence but also to the ability of a system to ignore details. When a state is the product of looking past or setting aside the multitude of variation, and it is also an instance of "gathering up an extended region of the flux and treating it as unity," then it is an instance of true intentionality.[73]

A similar idea can be found, I think, in Tyler Burge. According to Burge, perception is the most primitive kind of (non-deflated) representation, because it involves ignoring features of the proximal stimulus to give us what is distal and constant. Two features, in particular, are distinctive of perceptual representations as opposed to sensory states that merely track (in Burge's terminology 'register') information. One is that representations have veridicality conditions and appeal to their veridicality conditions plays a role in explanation. The other is objectification. This is the capacity of a perceptual state to depict a mind-independent and nonperspectival particular. Burge says:

> The kind representation constitutively involves capacities to represent veridically, and to have accuracy or veridicality conditions with non-trivial explanatory potential. The kind perception constitutively involves capacities to represent objectively—to represent some of the mind independent features of the environment veridically, as they are.
>
> (Burge 2010, p. 12)

According to Burge, registering states do not have these features:

> Some sensory information registration neither meets conditions for objectification nor has any constitutive or non-trivial explanatory association with veridicality conditions.
>
> (Burge 2010, p. 317)

73. Cantwell-Smith 1996, p. 226. Registration in Cantwell-Smith includes more than just perception (p. 192) and it is a distinctive mark of subjectivity, but I do not expand here on the differences between registration and perception in Cantwell-Smith.

What is telling is Burge's analysis of the motivations for counting internal structures of the perceptual system as having both veridicality conditions and the capacity for objectification. According to Burge, perceptual representations are subject to accuracy and error because they are the product of a process where *underdetermination* is resolved. In overcoming underdetermination, the visual system privileges certain possible distal causes of the stimulation over others.[74] In other words, states that are the product of ignoring and detaching from proximal ambiguity have accuracy conditions, thus also being genuine representations.

Early visual states, on the other hand, respond to the environment and may malfunction. They may malfunction in the sense of failing to fulfill their biological function, but they do not, according to Burge, privilege one cause over others in the same way. In studying them, we do not need to look for constrains, default settings or, what Burge calls, 'formation principles.' We can simply look at their response behavior to understand what they track. Registering states of this kind are not usefully viewed as truth-evaluable.[75] Truth-evaluability and representational status surface when a state is the result of solving underdetermination.

We see appeal to a similar idea, in Burge's analysis of how objectification is achieved in perception. Objectification, according to Burge, consists of overcoming the idiosyncratic aspects of the proximal stimulus to depict a mind-independent particular as having certain properties.[76] It is achieved by application of the perceptual constancies. Burge says:

> Perceptual constancies are capacities for objectification. Objectification separates registration of surface stimulation that is local to individual and occasion from elements in that registration that are (according to formation patterns) representationally specific to attributes in the physical environment. Thus objectification separates local, idiosyncratic registrations from representations of individual-independent, perspective-independent reality, beyond the individual.
>
> (Burge 2010, p. 399)

As we see in further detail in section 4.3, perceptual constancies are settings of the perceptual system that allow it to ignore variations in the proximal

74. Burge 2009, p. 315, 2010, pp. 344–345.

75. Burge 2010, pp. 301, 396.

76. Burge 2010, pp. 397–398.

stimulus in favor of constant distal conditions. One widely studied constancy applies to size. Despite variations in an object's retinal projection due to the observer moving closer and further away from it, we typically perceive objects as preserving size. This constancy allows the perceptual system to systematically neglect "aspects of sensory registration that are not likely to correlate with relevant environmental conditions" and to capitalize on aspects that are likely to correlate.[77] The constancies, according to Burge, enable the visual apparatus to "distinguish the merely proximal from the probably environmental."[78]

Burge is here suggesting that perceptual and representational states are distinctive for displaying objectification, and objectification occurs when there is some *distance* between the changing retinal stimulation and the percept. It is only when objectification is attained that we can talk of a state as representing a mind-independent particular. Representation, here, is of distal, relatively constant, elements.

If this is right, then there is an emerging consensus among those who reflect on the notion of representation. This consensus has it that representations are only those performance-guiding structures that are de-coupled from their causes, where this fact materializes in their standing for distal or absent conditions. In paradigmatic perceptual cases, representations do not encode certain aspects of the proximal stimulus—for example, its continuous variation—and, at the same time, reproduce features that are not present in the stimulus—for instance, its stability and hidden parts. In such cases, they are both about absent and distal conditions.

Thinking of representations this way respects their explanatory function and makes sense of our judgments. We are inclined to judge that the rabbit represents the coyote, because the rabbit's behavior is guided by states that stand for a whole, continuous animal, despite the fact that the stimulus to which the rabbit is exposed is both underdetermined and constantly changing.

Something similar can be said of the other examples we considered. If the frog represents at all, it does so because its inner states are about a whole, constant, and moving object, despite indeterminacy and variation in the stimulus. If, by contrast, we were able to explain the frog's behavior by thinking of it as simply tracking low-intensity light spots, then we should not think of its states in representational terms. Similarly, if a neural network stands for the hand-elbow-shoulder system, then it stands for something distal that abstracts

77. Burge 2010, pp. 397–398.

78. Ibid.

from the flux of proprioceptive feedback. Indeed, the capacity to respond to distal objects and properties marks a representational capacity even when the distal objects and properties are not as complex as coyotes or elbow-shoulder systems. When we see a line drawn on paper we also see something *distal*, because we see something constant and stable that preserves its appearance through changes in retinal projection.

For our overall project, this characterization of representational states has the consequence that only later stages of visual perception—the stages where completion, constancy, and stability have been achieved—are clearly representations. We may doubt, by contrast, that early visual states enjoy the same status. These states do not appear to have any effects on behavior, and they are too close to what causes them to occur. The boundary between these two kinds of states may be fuzzy, and the point where the visual process starts employing representations may be uncertain. The fact that there are unclear cases, however, should not discourage us from drawing the distinction in question. The distinction is needed and there are enough good examples of it.

To conclude, many subpersonal perceptual operations occur between tracking states. There may also be perceptual operations that occur between representational states. This, given our parameters, is ultimately an empirical question. In what follows, I argue that the extent to which this occurs has been largely exaggerated in vision research. There is a representation-inflation in this field. The suspicion is that, as Gibson supposes, vision is a cognitive process in highly artificial, experimental situations, where rich ambient information is absent—for example, the case of the Kanizsa triangle discussed in section 4.6. In those cases, the visual system may be forced to use states that stand for absent or distal elements, whereas in natural environments the system may simply respond (representationally) to external conditions without using any further representation. To show that this embedded way of looking at vision is empirically plausible, I now turn to the issue of evidence for both s- and p-representations.

3.6 The evidence: s-representations

The argument so far shows that EV is, on theoretical grounds, a plausible empirical hypothesis, as it is consistent with current reflection on the notion of representation, as well as with research in vision science. In this section, I begin to show that EV is also empirically plausible. If vision were mediated by representational states and structures, then we should find some evidence that indicates that it is. This is typically recognized by cognitivists themselves, who accept that they have an additional burden of proof.

This explanatory burden is particularly evident if we consider a committal view of representation. Holding that vision is mediated by representations in the committal sense means having some evidence to suppose that vision is mediated by map- or language-like states that serve as both s-representations and p-representations. It is far from clear, however, that early sensory states are representations, and it is even less clear that the visual apparatus needs map- or language-like structures that encode internalized principles of operation.[79]

Consider, first, sensory representations. Everyone—including non-cognitivists—can agree that the production of visual percepts is preceded by some sort of processing. Everyone can also agree that this processing happens in stages. The further question is whether we need to regard such stages as representational rather than as mere reliable intermediaries. The general tendency, however, is to suppose that admitting the stages is already committing to cognitivism. This is not right. Given what I argued so far, even if we found that the stages carried information by neatly and selectively co-varying with some environmental parameters—which is doubtful given predictive coding models—we would still have reason to wonder whether they act as representations.

This is evident if we remember the general idea that representations are performance-guiding states. One of the challenges is to show that intermediary structures have observable behavioral effects. This, however, is hard to do, it is rarely done, and when it is done it does not deliver the desired results.

Consider purported intermediaries of vision, such as retinal maps and the Marrian stages of visual processing. Retinal maps presumably reproduce the pattern of activation of retinal neurons. In so doing, they seem to display an interesting sort of isomorphism, but they are also close to their causal origin in a way that suggests that they simply track what they stand for. As far as I know, such maps do not inform behavior, let alone behavior in the absence of real-world feedback. Nothing seems to be lost by thinking of them as trackers—that is, by thinking of them in the same way in which we think of neurons that regulate optical muscle contraction.

---

79. In fact, the map-like view seems open to more general critiques of representational explanations of mental activity. A number of researchers point out that the creation of internal maps is an expensive process for an organism that has to interact smoothly with the environment. Such researchers remark that, in many cases, internal maps are neither needed nor useful to explain behavior. They would be an impediment to smooth performance (Beer 1995, Brooks 1991).

As we move up in the visual hierarchy from retinal maps, we presumably find states that stand for edges, lines, and surfaces. If we follow Marr's bottom-up theory, for example, we find a primal sketch consisting of representations of lines, edges, and blobs derived from the light reflected on the retina. Further up, we find a 21/2 D sketch where surfaces are represented in a subject-centered coordinate system.

Unlike retinal maps, states that stand for edges or surfaces have some distance from their causal origin, since they somewhat abstract from the variation of the stimulus present at the retina. The question still arises, however, as to whether these states exist, and as to whether we should think of them as representations. For one thing, Marr seemed inclined to posit such intermediate stages, at least in part, for theoretical reasons. He thought that it was necessary to break the problem of vision into steps to make it more tractable.[80] While this may be right, it *imposes* rather than *discovers* representational stages in vision. It imposes a well-defined hierarchical architecture that we may not find in biological visual systems.

Notice also that it is far from clear that the Marrian intermediaries have any behavioral effects. Indeed, if they are proprietary and insulated, we will not find this kind of evidence at all. What we find is that people's abilities are better explained by supposing that they represent not edges and surfaces in isolation but, rather, complete object-centered entities with stable boundaries. Supposing that people represent object-centered entities makes better sense, for example, of their spontaneous perceptual judgments concerning presented items.[81]

Significant, in this respect, is also a body of research on the perceptual capacities of infants and children. This research suggests that children and infants perceive the world in terms of rigid and persisting objects, not in terms of detached lines and surfaces. Infants at four months old expect objects to be solid, and to retain their spatio-temporal location when occluded. They are reliably surprised by the appearance of an object going through another object, or by the appearance of an object changing location without traveling some continuous path.[82] This research is taken to contradict Piaget's idea that the

---

80. Marr 1982, ch. 1.

81. Rosch et al. 1976. People are faster at naming and recognizing objects belonging to basic categories—for example, trees, cars, and chairs. Jerry Fodor uses these studies to argue that basic categories are the level of output of perceptual modules (Fodor 1983, pp. 93–94).

82. Baillargeon 1993, Spelke 1990, Xu and Carey 1996, Xu et al. 2004.

world of children is radically different from the world of adults in failing to contain persisting, three-dimensional entities.[83]

One may object that I am raising the bar too high. Subpersonal states of a system may not inform person-level behavior while also counting as representations. If our best model of a given mental capacity requires the existence of encapsulated states that stand for distal conditions, then such states are representations, even if they are only implicated in subpersonal operations.

While this may be a good point for mental representations in general, I think that it is useful to remember two points. First, in chapter 2, I introduced an approach to vision according to which percepts are created given the statistical relationship between retinal stimuli and their environmental causes. Diachronic perception is further explained by the brain's attempt to reduce error in the high-level percept by checking the activity of lower-level units. In this approach, while very low visual states may track proximal conditions—for instance, properties of light—it is not clear that the other stages stand for well-defined distal quantities. It is not clear, in particular, that we need well-specified Marrian stages to understand how visual percepts are generated.

This is evident if we think of modeling visual perception in a connectionist network, as predictive coding models do. It is hard to say what the units in a network encode, since such units respond in clusters—and in varying degrees—to all of the stimuli that come from input units. So, a plausible model of vision hardly dictates that we see intermediate stages as standing for identifiable distal conditions.

Further, I want to stress that I certainly did not come up with the idea that representations are performance-guiding states. This idea is commonly found in cognitive science. We need only look back at the examples from deflationists—frogs and bacteria. Consider also the following case from vision science involving amodal completion. This is one of the rare studies geared at testing precisely whether vision is mediated by intermediary representations.

---

83. Piaget 1999[1954]. This body of work can be used to support the view that children perceive the world similarly to adults, even if we take the work to be about the stages of *conceptual* development rather than about perception (Baillargeon 1993). Children and infants appear to have the concept of an object surprisingly early, making us suppose that the object-concept is primary when compared to other concepts (Sabo unpublished). This reading of the studies has obvious repercussions for perception, however. Perception is one important way in which humans acquire concepts. Plausibly, children have concepts of objects early because they perceive them. See also Orlandi 2010.

FIGURE 3.1 Occluded circle.

Amodal completion occurs when we perceive something that is not present to the senses but suggested by contextual factors as illustrated by figure 3.1. Observers typically report seeing a complete circle covered by a square, despite the fact that only a portion of the circle is visible. In cognitive accounts, the idea is that completion is achieved in representational stages, where the visual system first represents the fragments of the circle, and then completes it according to some discoverable principles.

Allison Sekuler and Stephen Palmer, wanting to defend a cognitive account, tried to find evidence for the role of intermediate representations in completion. They write:

> The issue of whether there are internal representations prior to completion is particularly important for perceptual theory because it bears critically on a central controversy between interpretive (Helmholtzian) and direct (Gibsonian) accounts of perception. According to interpretive accounts, there is an initial representation of the "proximal shape" that undergoes systematic development and elaboration from the moment the object is first seen until it is interpreted as a 3-D object in the world (cf. Marr, 1982; Rock, 1983). If so, it should be possible to find evidence of a two-dimensional (2-D) representation (a la Marr's "primal sketch" or Rock's "literal percept") very early in processing, prior to visual completion. According to direct accounts there is no such early representation from which the final percept is inferred. Perception consists of the extraction of invariants comprising the completed percept. This view predicts that one should find no evidence for an early 2-D representation prior to the completed, 3-D representation; indeed, the first and only representation one should find is that of a completed, 3-D figure.
>
> (Sekuler and Palmer 1992, p. 101)

In a series of ingenious experiments, Sekuler and Palmer tested the time course of completion together with their cognitive hypothesis. They used a priming paradigm to do so. When people are asked to make 'sameness judgments' concerning some presented shapes—that is, judgments of similarity concerning shapes—the time they take to make their responses is affected by a priming stimulus seen right before the shapes. For example, after seeing a complete circle, people are faster at saying 'same' to a pair of complete circles than to a pair of incomplete circles. By contrast, if people are primed with an incomplete circle—say, a pac–man figure—they are faster at judging that two incomplete circles are the same than at judging that two complete circles are the same. In short, complete circles prime complete circles and incomplete circles prime incomplete circles; similar shapes make the corresponding similarity judgments faster.

The question tested by Sekuler and Palmer is what happens when occluded shapes serve as primes. If occluded shapes prime complete figures, rather than incomplete ones, this indicates that subjects represent occluded figures as complete. This is in fact what was found. When subjects were primed with occluded circles—such as a circle partly covered by a square—they were faster at judging that two complete circles were the same than at judging that two incomplete circles were the same. This provides first-person independent reasons for the claim that occluded figures are represented as complete (figure 3.2).

Now, in explaining how the visual system forms a representation of a complete circle, cognitive accounts hold that such representation is the conclusion of a process where information is added to the representation of the fragments. This view predicts that we should find some evidence for the representation of the fragmented figure.

By further varying the time of priming—that is, the time of exposition to the prime—Sekuler and Palmer tested the time-course of completion and its stages. The idea is that, by varying the time to which a subject is exposed to the prime, we can uncover the behavior of the prime itself. If the exposition time is too low, and the occluded figure does not have a priming effect on the subsequent judgments, then we would have some evidence that completion is a process that extends in time, as well as some idea of how long it takes. If, in addition, we found that, with low exposition times, an occluded prime

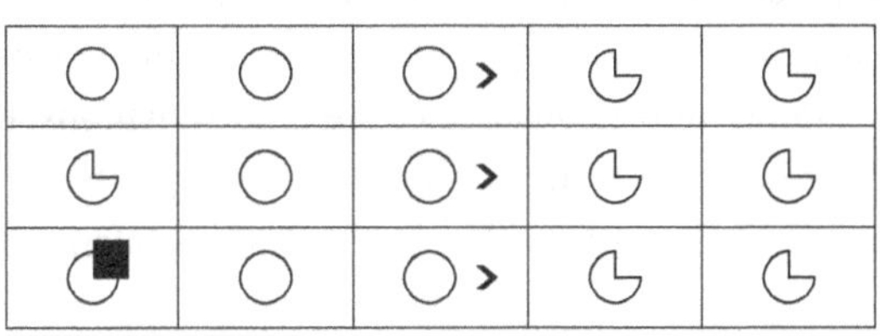

FIGURE 3.2 Priming effects on similarity judgments of complete, fragmented, and occluded figures.

behaved like a fragmented one—speeding judgments of similarity between incomplete figures—then we would have some evidence that occluded figures are first represented as fragmented. Using the priming paradigm can give us a snapshot of the process that underlies completion, as well as some sense of whether this process happens in representational stages.[84]

Despite what Sekuler and Palmer tentatively suggest, the results do not confirm the hypothesis that completion happens in representational steps, although they do confirm that completion takes time. The studies found that for long exposition times (400 ms) occluded primes behave almost identically to complete ones. They speed sameness judgments of complete figures and slow sameness judgments of incomplete ones. This confirms that occluded figures are perceived as complete.

Occluded and fragmented primes, however, do not produce virtually identical response times. For low exposition times, occluded primes do not consistently speed similarity judgments of incomplete figures. The evidence for expositions lower than 200 ms is, in fact, hard to judge, as 200 ms seems to be the limit for observing *any* priming effect. At 50 ms, for instance, complete circles did not prime complete circles judgments.

This study is a nice illustration of the idea that if observers represented occluded figures first as fragmented, then this should somehow show up in behavior. In this case, it should show up in the speed of similarity judgments between fragmented figures. Without this behavioral effect we would be unjustified in thinking that completion is achieved in representational stages.

The tacit assumption, in line with what I have been arguing, is that to show that perception is mediated by representations requires more evidence than the simple consideration that vision is usefully seen as stage-divided, or that it is mediated by states that respond to fragments. There may well be neurons that selectively track edges, lines, and other elements of the figure, yet this is deemed insufficient—even by cognitivists like Palmer—to prove that completion is due to an inferential process.

Checking for behavioral effects is a good way to check for the representational status of intermediary visual states. If the stages that precede completion, or stability, or the constancies are representations, then we should find observable evidence for their being so. Perhaps this means that the present section is to be read as a request for more evidence, rather than as

84. Sekuler and Palmer 1992, p. 101.

a definitive argument. It is such a request. Part of what I would like to achieve in this book is some sense of how to test competing empirical hypotheses in vision. We need some shared sense of how to test that a process is inferential, and that a state is representational. As far as I can see, given some plausible idea of what representations are, this evidence has not been offered for s-representations. The next section discusses whether the same can be said for p-representations. What evidence is there to suppose that visual systems represent their own principles of operation?

3.7 The evidence: p-representations

So far I argued that the tendency to view early vision as representing external conditions is poorly justified. Notice, however, that, even if it turned out that some intermediary visual states are representations, it would not follow that vision thereby also uses p-representations. Since encoding principles of perceptual processing is thought to be a precondition for deeming the visual process inferential, it would not follow that vision is inferential. Similarly, to grant that some low-level visual states are representations does not amount to granting that they are representations with propositional or linguistic structure. If one thinks that propositional structure is required for inference, then it would not follow that vision is inferential in this sense either. To further argue for an inferential account—given what has been said about inferences—we would need to also show that some principles of operation are encoded within perceptual systems. We would need to show that vision follows rules, rather than being a mere wired system.

Chapter 2 identified a few criteria for the ascription of p-representations. These criteria are generally mentioned by inferentialists themselves. One preliminary, but not conclusive, criterion consists of seeing what computational framework—if any—is more faithful in modeling a given system and reproducing its capacities. The idea is that there are different kinds of computers, some that plausibly follow rules, and some that simply act lawfully without encoding a rule. Depending on what kind of computer better models a biological system, we can get a preliminary indication of whether the system in question is of one type rather than the other.

For simplicity, we can frame this contrast in terms of the contrast between classical computers and connectionist networks. If classical digital computers provided the only model—or a much better model—of visual systems, then we would have some initial reason to suppose that vision is rule-following. However, the available research does not favor inferentialism in this respect.

While both digital computers and connectionist nets are not yet able to match the capabilities of biological visual systems, connectionists have been able to keep up with their more traditional competitors.

Artificial networks are famously good at pattern recognition, as they are capable of tolerating distortions and inexactness, and they learn from examples. Networks are typically able to learn to pick up on, and to recognize, entities that deviate incrementally from some prototype. This has proven handy when it comes to building artifacts that can see. Connectionist machines can be programmed to achieve color constancy and to detect a number of environmental inputs including faces and their gender, facial expressions, head orientation, complex shapes, and objects from images.[85] It follows that the first criterion for proving that visual operations follow encoded rules does not favor the inferentialist. Wired computational systems are able to replicate some central visual competences.

There are two additional criteria for judging that a system follows rules, and these criteria do not make reference to computational models. They rather diagnose the presence of represented principles from the behavior and capacities of a system, thus abstracting from how the system is built. According to the first of these two additional criteria, a system represents a rule when the rule is used and available in a number of contexts. In paradigmatic intelligent systems—like human cognizers—a rule may be available to higher thought and figure in the cognizer's belief set.

This criterion emerges from reflecting on the difference between systems that intuitively represent principles and systems that do not. Humans are typically able to recount the rule they followed in exhibiting a certain behavior, or to mention the principle that regulated the drawing of a certain inference. In wired systems, by contrast, the rules that they conform to do not appear anywhere else in the performance of the system.

According to this criterion, in order to see whether visual systems follow rules, we should ask whether the assumptions that supposedly regulate them are found somewhere else in the cognitive architecture—for instance, in the observer's belief stock or in memory.

When we apply this criterion, however, we end up having little reason to suppose that the assumptions are encoded. This is because visual assumptions are proprietary to visual processing. They only apply within visual

85. Grossberg 1993, O'Toole and Abdi 1989, Plebe and Domenella 2007, Rae and Ritter 1998, Rosenblum et al. 1996, Sabisch et al. 2000, Stanikunas et al. 2004, Zhang and Fulcher 1996.

systems to a restricted set of stimuli, and they are not available to any process outside the visual system.[86] Observers do not know what the assumptions are, prior to doing vision science.

In this context, a clarification is in order. In describing inferential accounts in previous chapters, I simplified the formulation of the assumptions that supposedly regulate visual processing. I said, for example, that representations of edges are derived from representations of discontinuities in light intensity, and from the assumption that edges are the typical causes of such discontinuities. Similarly, I said, in a simplistic fashion, that the visual system arranges surfaces into three-dimensional objects by following the rule that surfaces inhere in them. This may give the impression that the principles employed by the visual apparatus are present in our belief set. We do believe that surfaces inhere in three-dimensional objects.

My formulation was, however, a simplification used for expository purposes. The rules to which visual processing conforms are more complicated and technical than what I said. The spatial coincidence assumption, for example, reads as follows:

> If a zero-crossing segment is present in a set of independent channels over a contiguous range of sizes and the segment has the same position and orientation in each channel, then the set of such zero-crossing segments may be taken to indicate the presence of an intensity change in the image that is due to a single physical phenomenon (a change in reflectance, illumination, depth or surface orientation). (. . .) It follows (. . .) that provided the two channels are reasonably separated in the frequency domain, and their zero-crossings agree, the combined zero-crossings can be taken to indicate the presence of an edge in the image.
>
> (Marr and Hildreth 1980, p. 202)

The principles regulating perception are discovered by researchers studying human perceptual capacities. They are not known by ordinary observers. Similarly, the laws of the empirical sciences—such as, the laws of physics—are discovered and not known by ordinary people.[87]

86. Pylyshyn 1999, pp. 344 and 356.

87. Appeal to Gestalt psychology provides no help in this context. According to Gestaltists, perception is regulated by rules of simplicity, proximity, symmetry, similarity and closure. These rules are coherent with the rest of our knowledge, and they may also show up in conscious thought. We perceive occluded objects as complete because such completion 'makes

If this is right, and perceptual principles are proprietary, then the second criterion for judging that they are encoded within visual systems is not met. We still lack grounds for thinking of biases as representational features.

Help for the cognitivist may come from a final criterion. This is the idea that systems that follow rules are, other things being equal, sensitive to evidence that runs contrary to the rules themselves.[88] The thought is that rule-following organisms are capable of adjusting to contrary information in a way that wired systems are not able to do. This criterion emerges, again, from reflecting on the intuitive difference between the two types of systems. People appear to be sensitive to evidence that renders their own principles of inference invalid. If one has evidence that, in a given context, a rule of inference is not truth-conducive, then one is—at least sometimes—capable of refraining from applying it. This capacity is diagnostic of the fact that one represents the rules that regulate one's actions.

Wired systems, on the other hand, do what they do regardless of whether or not they have evidence that runs at odds with the principles to which they conform. They do what they do somewhat blindly. They are not sensitive to the fact that, in some contexts, what they do may not be truth- or survival-conducive. This is, in fact, widely acknowledged as a hallmark of associative systems, as opposed to inferential ones. Associative systems are not reason-responsive.

Accordingly, the final proposal is that we could count some principles as represented—and a transition or a process as inferential—if a given system appeared to be sensitive to evidence. *Vice versa*, if a system is associative or wired, then it should not be reason-responsive.

When we apply this criterion, however, we are again led to conclude that the principles of operation are not encoded within visual systems. This is

---

sense', and accords with the rest of our knowledge about objects (Kanizsa 1985, Koffka 1935, Wertheimer 1923). In effect, however, the specific rules that describe how visual elements are grouped together, or how important symmetry is when compared to other factors, are more complicated than the Gestaltists first supposed (Pylyshyn 1999, p. 345, Wagemans et al. 2012). Even if such rules, in some sense, cohere with the rest of our knowledge, they are not part of people's belief sets prior to doing cognitive psychology. They are discovered by cognitive scientists.

88. The qualification 'other things being equal' is important. To show that a process is not reason-responsive is not thereby to show that it is not inferential. An *irrational* process is not thereby an *a-rational* process. It could be that the inferences are insulated from contrary evidence (Mandelbaum unpublished). While this may be true, we would then need other motivations to suppose that the process in question is indeed inferential. I have been arguing that, in the visual case, we lack other motivations.

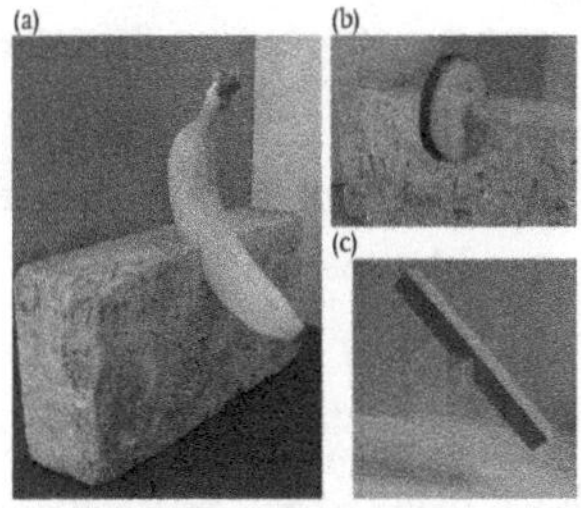

FIGURE 3.3 Insensitivity to reason in completion. From Gerbino and Zabai 2003.

because such systems appear to be insensitive to contrary information. Perceptual illusions, such as the Müller-Lyer illusion, are famous examples of this fact. The illusions persist despite our knowledge that they are illusory. If vision were sensitive to contrary information, then knowledge of the illusion should, *ceteris paribus*, change the way we see it. That this is not the case indicates that the idea that visual systems are wired is a live option.[89]

Examples of the stubbornness of vision are given even outside the realm of perceptual illusions. The visual system appears to be insensitive to evidence in the case of amodal completion as well. Figures and objects are often completed in ways that seem odd if one considers contextual information. figure 3.3 illustrates this point. Given our knowledge of the material objects depicted in figure 3.3, we should be able to change how the image looks. Since hard materials (the brick) are hard to penetrate, we should be able to easily perceive the banana and the eggplant as incomplete. This is generally not the case, however. Most perceivers report seeing them as whole, despite evidence that runs contrary to this interpretation. Acknowledging the evidence does nothing to change how the elements of the figure appear. Similarly, in figure 3.3(c) observers report a sense of completeness of the bar despite perceiving a transparent box. The perceptual process that leads to completion seems to be unaffected by conflicting information.[90]

What is noteworthy in these cases, is that there seems to be a very clear separation between what we perceive and what we know to be the case, where the latter does not affect the former. How things look seems preset, and impervious to known inconsistencies suggesting that vision is wired and autonomous.

89. More on this in sections 4.5 and 4.8.

90. Gerbino and Zabai 2003, Kanizsa 1979, Kanizsa and Gerbino 1982.

In response to these considerations, inferentialists can appeal to the perceived *plasticity* of visual perception. This plasticity generally comes in two forms that are often discussed together.[91] First, vision displays a certain amount of *flexibility*, being able to adapt to both physiological and environmental changes. Second, vision is said to be *cognitively penetrable*, or influenced by other psychological states. Multi-stability (see section 4.7) is sometimes indicated as an example of cognitive penetrability, but I give more examples of penetrability in section 4.8, where I argue that instances of cognitive penetration are not instances where the visual system is reason-responsive.

To conclude this section and chapter, I want to look at the *flexibility* of the visual system. Such flexibility can be mistaken for a sign of rule-following. To address this mistake, I briefly argue that the flexibility of vision does not point to its inferential nature, and it is compatible with the visual apparatus being embedded.

Adaptable wired systems

The adaptability of vision in response to physiological and environmental changes is sometimes taken as an indication that the visual system is not wired. The reason for this is that the term 'wired' is often used interchangeably with 'hardwired'; both are taken to be synonyms of 'immutable.'[92] Irvin Rock, for example, appeals to the malleability of vision to argue in favor of inferentialism. He points out that the visual system may come to conform to a different rule, or set of rules. He writes:

> (. . .) we can conclude that a new rule can be acquired and govern perception. The fact that such rules can be learned and then determine perception is very convincing evidence that they are internally represented.
>
> (Rock, 1983, p. 277)

To support his claim, Rock gives the example of wearing inverting lenses.[93] Normally, vision conforms to a rule that allows it to ignore the changing retinal projection caused by a stationary object. When our heads move, the image

91. Churchland 1989.

92. Goldstone 2003, p. 234.

93. Rock 1983, p. 276, Stratton 1896.

projected by an unmoving entity sweeps over the retina in a particular direction and at a particular rate. The visual system must take this into consideration and conform to a principle that may be roughly the following:

> Image displacement to the right at *x* degrees per second during head rotation to the right at *x* degrees per second implies that the objects imaged are stationary.
>
> (Rock 1983, p. 276)

This principle regulates vision in normal circumstances, but the visual system can come to conform to a different principle when the subject wears inverting lenses. The lenses reverse the direction of image displacement during head motion. At first, the scene appears to rotate in the direction of head movements. This is because the relationship between image displacement and head rotation no longer holds as it did without the lenses. After some time, the visual system adapts to the new situation and subjects are able to see the world normally. This is taken as evidence that the visual apparatus has now acquired a new rule. This, in turn, is supposed to show that the new rule is encoded and followed in the computation.

I think that this is a mistake. The fact that vision can come to operate differently from how it is set to operate is no reason to suppose that it encodes principles.

To see why this is the case, consider that systems that are wired in our sense show adaptiveness and malleability of the kind described. Connectionist and neural networks are a prime example of this fact. Networks are wired systems capable of adjusting to context. In the learning period, they come to process information in a new way without having any localizable structures that encode instructions. They come to be sensitive to the presence of mine echoes by simply adjusting their connections. Similarly, pigeons may stop pecking on a key as a result of extinction or counterconditioning without following any rules.

Associative and wired systems are capable of changing their performance. This happens when environmental or physiological interventions disrupt the associations they instantiate. The fact that they are adaptable in this way does not mean that they are rule-following. Rewiring due to inverting lenses, or to reinforcement and reward, amounts to changing the way a certain function is performed through a physical intervention. It constitutes an instance of malleability without being an instance of following (new) principles.

For a familiar analogy, consider that we could rewire smoke detectors and change their mode of processing. Suppose that we wired a detector so that it responded to more elements than just to the presence of smoke. Perhaps we could introduce a metallic strip within the system so that, given the expansion of the strip with temperature, the detector was able to pick up on heat. Heat is also a good indicator of fire in the environment. By doing this, we would cause the alarm to be a better sensor of fire, but we wouldn't do so in virtue of introducing a new rule. We would rather do so in virtue of manipulating some functional feature of the alarm.

In biological systems, this manipulation can be due to environmental or physiological pressure—for instance, wearing lenses—rather than to the work of a designer. The result is analogous. The biological system may come to adjust to new circumstances through a physical reconfiguration, sometimes in advantageous ways.

We should then resist the tendency to suppose that flexibility is always a sign of rule-following, and that 'wired,' 'hardwired,' and 'immutable' go together. Flexibility is a sign of rule-following only if it is also an instance of reason-responsiveness. In the visual case, inverting lenses simply cause a rewiring of the visual system—that is, the weakening of some connections and strengthening of others—thus constituting a fairly unconsequential case of flexibility. Indeed, even outside the perceptual domain, it seems clear that systems that are constrained and associative have a certain degree of malleability.[94] To think of a wired system as immutable seems to be an instance of the dubious dichotomy between nature and nurture, as if wired systems were incapable of changing their performance given context.[95]

Equally as problematic, in this context, is the equation of 'wired' with 'innate.' To suppose that a system is wired is not thereby to suppose that the way it functions is specified innately, or at birth. A system may come to be wired to function in a certain way as a result of environmental pressure. How it functions need not be specified 'in the genes.'[96]

94. Sea slugs do not represent the principles that regulate their retractive and defensive behavior. Yet they are also somewhat adaptive and flexible, being subject to both habituation—the progressive decrease in response to a repeated stimulus—and sensitization—the increase in response due to the presentation of a novel stimulus. See Frank and Greenberg 1994.

95. Thanks to James Campbell for making this point explicit.

96. Thanks to an anonymous referee for making this issue explicit.

This is a point that I tried to stress in my characterization of the embedded view. Thinking of the visual system as embedded means thinking of it as a system that, under environmental pressure—in the evolutionary past *and in the present*—develops physical features that make it process inputs in a certain way. The environmental pressure on embedded visual systems is *ongoing*. It comes from the specific environment that surrounds each of us. Under such pressure, vision can come to develop new features, and to process information differently, without thereby encoding any principles.

This explains why 'experience'—intended as prior exposure, rather than as phenomenological experience—affects the way we see. Exposure to a given environment influences the way we see because it influences how the visual apparatus is set to process information. A number of studies suggest, for example, that observers in 'carpentered worlds' are more prone to geometrical illusions (such as the Müller-Lyer) than subjects exposed to noncarpentered worlds.[97] A carpentered environment is one where geometrical figures and structures abound. Given such environments, we can expect visual systems to be wired to process input more geometrically, and to be wired differently in places where right angles and straight lines are not as common.[98]

If this is true, then that a system can come to conform to new principles does not show either that the system follows rules or that the system is sensitive to contrary evidence and capable of adjusting to it. Visual systems are malleable and yet embedded.

To conclude, we should briefly recap this section. We started with three criteria for judging that a system encodes its own principles of operation. One criterion concerns what computational model better reproduces the system's capacities. The second criterion is about whether the principles are widely available for the performance of other tasks. The third, and final, criterion concerns whether the system appears sensitive to evidence that runs at odds with the principles. I argued that, according to these criteria, visual systems are best seen as constrained and embedded. I argued further that showing that the systems are adaptable is no reason to think that they follow rules.

---

97. Ahluwalia 1978. I leave aside, here, the issue of whether the studies are reliable. I aim to show that, *if* they are, they can be explained in an embedded framework.

98. Accordingly, we may also see the world differently compared to our evolutionary ancestors as a function of inhabiting different environments. Thanks to Kranti Saran for pressing this issue.

3.8 Conclusion

This chapter argued that constraints are different from implicit representations, and that deflationary notions of representation misunderstand the notion. The chapter provided a positive proposal for what representations are. Both the proposal and the distinctions defended here are not mere philosophical sophistications. They respect the function that representations play in explanation. They are found in a number of areas of the cognitive sciences, as well as in the work of a number of researchers who otherwise disagree. They reflect an emerging consensus on the notion of representation.

In sections 3.6 and 3.7, I further argued that, given this shared understanding of representational structures, we lack evidence for supposing that the states and features that mediate vision are representations. Cognitivism is not supported by the evidence. This provides reasons to prefer the embedded view. EV emerges as a more plausible, and better justified, account of visual perception. The next chapter is devoted to showing that it is also explanatorily powerful.

4

The explanatory power of the Embedded View

I am vastly oversimplifying the situation. There are many types of transition between sensory states in a perceptual system, whether the states are both nonperceptual, one is nonperceptual and the other is perceptual, or both are perceptual. An adequate feel for the science requires direct exposure to it.

(BURGE 2009, p. 316 n. 57)

4.1 Introduction

If the embedded view is right, then vision is naturally constrained to produce representations from states that are merely sensitive and respond in various ways to environmental situations. I argued for the plausibility of this view by claiming that it better accords with contemporary research in vision science and with reflection on the notion of representation. EV respects the explanatory function that representations are called to perform. In light of this plausibility, the further challenge is to show that the embedded view has explanatory power. Inferential and interpretive accounts are often preferred to competing accounts—for example, Gibsonian alternatives—because they are said to explain a variety of visual phenomena that are otherwise mysterious.

This chapter is devoted to providing embedded models of visual cases that pose difficulties for direct views. What is crucial is to recognize that the embedded view does not hold that no processing at all happens between retinal stimulation and the production of visual percepts. EV only holds that such processing does not consist in an inference.

This is an important point because ecological views of perception are often taken to claim that no relevant explanatory advantage comes from looking at the internal complexity of perceptual systems. By contrast, I think that it is open to such views to admit functional complexity without thereby committing to any more inflated representational claim.

This chapter starts by reiterating briefly how the embedded view accounts for the stability of vision and then sketches explanations of other relevant visual cases. The chapter is roughly divided into two parts. In the first part, I look at instances where vision appears to be quite inflexible and wired. In constancy, misperception, illusion, and completion the visual system appears to process information in a set and hardly changeable way. Visual cases of this kind may be particularly apt to being explained in an embedded framework. In the second part of the chapter, I look at cases where vision appears to be malleable and to be subject to some measure of control. Perhaps these are better examples for the cognitivist as the flexibility of perception may be taken as a sign of its inferential nature.

In this second part, I offer an embedded account of multi-stability, the phenomenon where the same figure or object is seen in multiple ways and, in section 4.8, I discuss occurrences of cognitive penetrability. Visual perception is cognitively penetrable when what we see is affected not just by external stimuli or viewing conditions, but by other psychological states, such as beliefs. In such cases, what one sees depends on, and changes with, one's knowledge and expertise. Cognitivists may appeal to cases of cognitive penetrability to demonstrate that the visual apparatus is reason-responsive and not wired. I show, by contrast, that penetrability is compatible with EV. Embedded visual systems are as flexible as penetrability requires.

Two final points about this chapter: some of the sections to follow provide a bit of history of how a given phenomenon has been explained in the past. Most of the sections outline an inferential explanation first, and the embedded alternative emerges contrastively. In proposing the alternative, I do not mean to provide a complete account of the visual cases in question. For each of the cases, there may be more that needs to be said to explain their ontogenesis and phenomenology. As long as this would be true of *any* model of visual processing—embedded or inferential—I will be content with giving the beginning of a story. My aim is to simply show that insofar as an inferential outlook can explain these different visual cases, an embedded outlook can also do so. In fact, in many instances, the embedded outlook accords better with the empirical evidence.

Further, the list of visual phenomena presented here is not exhaustive. It includes instances that seem particularly troubling for direct accounts. There may be cases, however, that I am not covering, and that are better treated in an inferential framework. As already admitted, this is how it should be since whether vision is embedded is ultimately an empirical question. This chapter is intended primarily to provide a strategy for non-inferentialists. The aim is to propose a non-inferential way of treating visual cases that can be applied to novel instances.

4.2 Stability

By this point in the book, it should be relatively clear what the fact of stability is. The pattern of light that hits the retina is fundamentally underdetermined—that is, compatible with a number of distal scenes. If vision were a direct response to the stimulus, then it seems that we should see the world in a radically unstable way—that is, we should flip back and forth between different perceptions of the same distal configuration. This is patently false, however. We see stable items that do not change their appearance (much) over time. So, vision is not direct.

Explaining stability in an embedded framework means recognizing that there is mediation in vision but that this mediation is not of the representational kind. So vision can be mediated while also being direct and non-inferential. We only need to think of the visual system as biased by environmental contingencies and as sensitive to environmental conditions.[1]

To use our usual example, discontinuities in light intensity at the retina can *in principle* be caused by edges, cracks, shadows, and many other environmental conditions. Suppose, however, that *in practice*—that is, in our specific environment—edges are the normal causes of light discontinuities—something that is within the purview of Natural Scene Statistics to study. Or, suppose that even if edges are not more frequent than shadows, it is a fact about us as biological organisms that they are more important to detect than other entities. Then we can expect the visual apparatus to be constrained to form hypotheses about edges—that is, to form states that respond to them.

This would mean that neural units that track light discontinuities activate units that track edges because this has proven accurate (or advantageous) in the past. The transition between these two tracking states is not regulated by an encoded assumption. We can think of it as a mere associative transition. What is relevant is that there is a strong connection between states that track discontinuities in intensity and states that track edges. This connection is a functional feature that evolved because of the regularity

1. In an article that criticizes direct accounts of perception, and that I discuss in some further detail in secion 4.4, Jerry Fodor and Zenon Pylyshyn remark that inference and direct 'pick-up' exhaust the psychological processes that could produce perceptual knowledge (Fodor and Pylyshyn 1981, p. 141). If by 'pick-up' they mean a process that is not mediated by functional states, then I disagree that the two mechanisms they identify exhaust the possibilities.

between discontinuities and edges (or because of the advantage). The system that picks up on edges acts in a way that is lawful and so describable by principles, but it does so in virtue of non-representational elements.

The type of picture I just sketched seems to be all that we need to explain stability. Given the incidence and importance of edges in the world, the visual system tracks them rather than something else, and does so consistently despite the fact that the incoming stimulation is compatible with other distal causes. Indeed it would be surprising if it were otherwise. Given the ubiquitousness and importance of edges, it would be surprising if evolution did not take care of this. In this explanation, external facts account for why we pick up on edges rather than on something else. No additional representational resources are needed.

Similarly, at later stages of visual processing—where representations are more plausibly involved—vision forms representations of three-dimensional objects in response to tracking surfaces, not because of any internal knowledge but because it is wired to do so. Presumably, it is important for us to see three-dimensional objects, and it is further plausible that, in our environment, surfaces with certain characteristics typically inhere in them. These facts are explanatory of our perceptual capacities.

In this picture, we recognize, in Gibsonian spirit, the richness of the stimulus that hits the eye. This richness is present in the form of the statistical regularities between visual input and distal causes. The richness, together with considerations of utility, ultimately explains why we see a *stable* world. The additional idea, from the predictive coding literature, that the brain is primarily concerned with reducing error is not central to explaining how the inverse problem is solved, and how stability is achieved. The 'driving signal' makes sense of how we arrive at a single percept (see section 2.4). The attempt to reduce error does account, however, for how a stable percept is *maintained* once it is formed. Bayesian models of perceptual activity—understood in noncommittal terms—describe and explain *diachronic* aspects of perception—for instance, how a percept is maintained and how it may change over time. As a consequence, an embedded account of visual processing has little trouble explaining stability.

4.3 Constancy

The fact of perceptual constancy is often discussed together with the fact of stability and used to introduce the idea that vision is inferential.[2] This

2. Rock 1983.

makes it appear as though constancy and stability are essentially the same phenomenon. Although, in both cases, vision ignores certain features of proximal stimulation, it is useful to keep these two phenomena separate.

Constancy poses the following problem. Because our retinas are located on moving eyes, heads, and bodies, and because environmental light conditions constantly change, the retinal stimulation is continuously changing. It follows that the light projected from an object is likely to vary from moment to moment. If there were a direct correlation between the light reflected and the percepts we experience, then we would perceive objects as continuously changing in certain important properties—for example, in color and size. We do not, however. We tend to perceive them as preserving most of their properties.[3]

As a first example, consider brightness. As we saw in section 2.3, the light reflected by a surface changes greatly as a function of illumination. An achromatic surface (a black, white, or gray wall) reflects light much differently if it is illuminated by a lamp or by sunlight, and different parts of the wall reflect light differently as a function of shadows. Yet, despite this variation, we are typically able to see white walls in houses and other buildings as having roughly the same lightness all over.

Like in the case of stability, the visual system is here called to solve a problem. It needs to distinguish adventitious features of retinal stimulation from features that correspond to entities in the world. While stability concerns primarily picking a single cause over the many that could have originated the stimulus, constancy is about ignoring the fluctuating aspects of the stimulus in favor of a homogeneous property. In lightness constancy, for instance, we have to make sense of how we perceive objects as uniformly light (or dark) despite variation in the light they reflect both synchronically and diachronically.

Early explanations of lightness constancy appealed to the constant ratios of adjacent surfaces.[4] Although different surfaces may reflect light differently at different times, the ratio of the intensity of light they reflect remains constant. A white surface reflects more intense light than a gray one, even if the amount of light they individually reflect varies from moment to moment. The idea is to explain brightness constancy by supposing that the perceived lightness is a

---

3. Vision scientists tend to assume perceptual constancy. Phenomenological considerations may put this assumption into question by showing, for example, that walls illuminated differently appear colored differently. In this section, I am not interested in disputing the truth of the assumption. I am interested, instead, in whether EV is capable of explaining the constancies, once we assume them.

4. Wallach 1948.

function of the constant ratios of reflected light, rather than a function of the varying illumination of a single surface.

To account for instances in which a single surface is present, and no comparison with a nearby surface is available, this theory is often integrated with a more general inferential approach to brightness constancy.[5] In inferential frameworks, the visual system achieves constancy by *assuming* that certain changes must be ignored. One assumption that is particularly important in this context is that only those discontinuities in light intensity that are sharp, and not blurry or fuzzy, are caused by reflectance changes.[6]

This implicit assumption reflects the fact that shadows in our environment do not have very sharp boundaries on a surface. The presence of a blurry contour points to a mere change in illumination, while a sharp contour indicates the presence of a more radical change—that is, a change in brightness. This explains why certain light discontinuities at the retina—those that are blurry—are simply ignored by the visual system and dismissed as illumination changes.

It is clear, however, that an embedded explanation is also available for this type of constancy. Assuming that perceiving brightness is important for creatures like us, and given the fact that blurry discontinuities are typically caused by shadows rather than by changes in color, we can expect visual systems to respond to blurry discontinuities with states that stand for brightness-invariant surfaces. The environmental fact that only certain discontinuities matter put its stamp on vision by skewing it to ignore certain other discontinuities (the blurry ones). The presence of a blurry intensity change in the stimulus is processed to produce a color invariant percept, and, once the perceptual hypothesis is that a surface is the same color all over, the presence of blurry contours at the retina produces no error signal.

In this explanation, what is crucial for understanding the constancies is again studying the environmental conditions that give rise to a given stimulus—for example, what conditions give rise to blurry contours at the retina. By studying such conditions vision scientists are able to predict what subjects experience without needing to think of vision as assuming anything (implicitly or explicitly) about the conditions themselves.[7]

---

5. Thanks to Todd Ganson for this point.

6. Burge 2010, p. 353, Palmer 1999, p. 132. See also Rock 1983, p. 276 for the idea that, in achieving constancy, vision makes use of *assumptions*.

7. See Nundy and Purves 2002 for a more detailed treatment of brightness constancy.

We can (very briefly) put this approach to work to explain another popular constancy, the one pertaining to size. The size of an object's retinal image varies not only as a function of the actual size of an object but also depending on its distance from the viewer. Objects that are further away project a smaller patch on the retina than objects that are close by. If there were a direct correlation between the retinal image and the perceived dimensions of an object, we would experience items as consistently changing in size. We do not. In ordinary circumstances, we perceive objects as preserving their dimensions regardless of their distance. This is the fact of size constancy.

Inferential accounts seem well-poised to explain size constancy because they ascribe to vision some implicit assumptions concerning size and its relation to distance.[8] Roughly, the visual system 'knows' that objects do not change in size as their distance changes. So, having represented an increase in distance, the system enlarges the size of an object to retain size constancy.[9]

The relationship between distance and perceived size is actually a bit more complicated and non-linear than this simple rendition suggests.[10] What matters, however, is the gist of the account provided by inferential outlooks. The idea is, again, that some internal assumptions are used to derive constant percepts from unstable and changing stimuli.

Yet again, an embedded alternative explanation is readily available. The key is to suppose that whatever facts are encoded inside are, instead, responsible for wiring the visual system to act in a certain way. Given that, in our world, size does not change with distance, we can expect the visual apparatus

---

8. Palmer 1999, p. 315, Rock 1983, p. 279.

9. Here are a couple of quotes that illustrate this way of explaining size constancy. Irvin Rock says:

> I will argue that the process of achieving constancies is one of deductive inference where the relevant "premises" are immediately known. That is to say, in the case of a specific constancy, such as that of size, two aspects of the proximal stimulus are most relevant, one being the visual angle subtended by the object and the other being information about the object's distance. The executive agency "knows" that these are the relevant aspects and therefore proceeds to relate them to one another.
>
> (Rock 1983, p. 240)

He adds:

> It is well known that size perception is intimately related to distance perception. Perceived size is a function not of the object's visual angle alone but of the distance at which the object is perceived to be as well.
>
> (Rock 1983, p. 249)

10. Epstein et al. 1961.

to be wired to respect this fact.[11] Variations in tracked distance activate states that enlarge the size of an object to retain size constancy. Constancy, just like stability, is thus readily explained in a direct and embedded framework.

4.4 Misperception

In a famous critical article concerning Gibsonian and direct accounts of vision, Jerry Fodor and Zenon Pylyshyn remark that an adequate account of perception has to be an account of perceptual error.[12] While it is easy to see how error takes place if visual processing is inferential, it is not as easy to see how Gibsonian alternatives explain error. If vision were direct, shouldn't we always see the world correctly? The fact that we do not is problematic.

Fodor and Pylyshyn suggest that inferentialism stands at an advantage compared to competitors because misperception is connected to failed inferences. They write:

> Your perception that something is edible, for example, is said to depend upon inferences from the appearance of the thing (e.g. from its smell, taste, texture, shape, color, and so forth). These inferences depend upon generalizations gleaned from past experience, and the generalizations are themselves nondemonstrative and hence fallible. So, for these and other reasons, the (perceptual) inference from appearance to edibility sometimes goes wrong, with consequences that are typically painful and occasionally fatal.
>
> (Fodor and Pylyshyn 1981, p. 153)

In line with Fodor and Pylyshyn, Irvin Rock remarks that the occurrence of error is convincing evidence for the existence of represented rules within the visual apparatus;[13] and contemporary *opponents* of inferential visual systems concede that misperception is a problem for their position. Ron McClamrock, for example, says:

> The intuitive argument against direct perception is a simple one: the argument from illusion—or, if you like, the "dominance of the proximal." You can have the percept without having the object as long as

11. See Howe and Purves 2005b, ch. 5.

12. Fodor and Pylyshyn 1981.

13. Rock 1983, p. 279.

> you have the right proximal stimulus; but you can't have the percept without the right proximal stimulus, even if you do have the object.
>
> (McClamrock 1995, p. 140)[14]

By reflecting on the embedded view, however, we should be able to see that the stress on inferences to explain misperception is a red herring. What is required for misperceiving is not that percepts are produced through inferences. What is required is rather that, first, percepts are states that are assessable for accuracy; and, second, that percepts are produced with some sort of causal mediation. Gibsonian accounts have trouble explaining misperception when they deny that visual states are states that have content, and when they downplay the functional mediation that is needed to produce them. Their problem is not that they hold vision to be direct, in the sense of not being inferential. Embedded models that think of percepts as representational states, and admit a causal process to generate them, have no trouble explaining how misperception takes place.

The key move is to think that the visual system is biased (as a result of environmental pressure) to prefer certain distal causes to others. This makes the system susceptible to error. Using our usual example, vision is constrained to prefer edges rather than shadows when exposed to discontinuities in light intensity of a certain kind. Being so constrained, the visual system is prone to sometimes get things wrong. Discontinuities in light intensity of a certain kind can be caused by shadows too, and when they are, they fool vision into signaling the wrong thing.

Indeed error can occur even in non-inferential mechanisms that use only tracking states, as long as we are willing to regard such states as having some sort of accuracy conditions. Recall smoke detectors. They rely on the environmental regularity that smoke particles deflect light particles to detect the presence of smoke. Smoke particles, however, are not the only particles that can interfere with the path of light in the detector's optical chamber. Vapor and gas can also do that. Thus smoke detectors can signal the presence of smoke even when vapor and gas are present. Indeed, if one were to intentionally deviate the beam of light to hit the sensor, perhaps by using a mirror, the detector could be tricked into signaling the presence of smoke in the absence of smoke

14. Interestingly, the 'argument from illusion' is also traditionally offered in favor of sense-data theory (Ayer 1967, Price 1950, p. 27). In chapter 1, section 1.4 I noted some rough similarities between contemporary inferentialism and sense-data theory but I will not expand on the similarities here.

or any other gas. If we suppose that detectors do not perform any inferences, then we are conclude that inferences are not needed to explain error.

In general, a system that uses causal or functional mediators to signal or represent a given quantity is susceptible to error. One only needs to activate the mediators to produce the signal without the distal cause. If there is little reason to think of the mediators as representations—like I think it is the case in vision—then we can explain misperception without appeal to any inferential process.

As a matter of fact, inferentialists would have to concede this point since they also think that some sensory representations—and thus some states that are capable of inaccuracy—are produced without inferences. Some representations are produced by mechanisms of transduction—that is, mechanisms that convert a physical property into an energy impulse (e.g., a neuronal reaction).[15] So the problem with Gibsonian views is not that they are not inferential. The problem for such views arises if they deny that vision produces states that are capable of being accurate or inaccurate, and if they understate the importance of causal intermediaries in vision. In this case, it is hard to see how a perceiving organism could misperceive.

Curiously, Fodor and Pylyshyn, despite the inferential rhetoric, should find the embedded way of understanding misperception (and perception) likable. Fodor and Pylyshyn often talk of early visual states not as representations but as detectors.[16] Such states being produced by transducers, are about properties of light—for example, intensity and wavelength—rather than properties of the layout. Detectors constitute the *specifiers* for the perception of the layout where that means that the perception is *causally* dependent on the sensory states.[17] This way of describing early vision, however, casts doubt on whether early visual states are representations—and on whether perception is inferential—for two reasons.

First, the relevant relation between sensory states so described and percepts is causal. It is not clear why, on top of being causal, it also needs to be semantic or 'epistemic' (as Fodor and Pylyshyn remark that it should be). Early visual states, in this case, do not appear to be informants in any relevant sense.[18] Second, given what they detect, thinking of sensory states as

15. Fodor and Pylyshyn 1981, p. 158, Pylyshyn 1984, ch. 6.

16. See, for example, Fodor and Pylyshyn 1981, p. 162.

17. Fodor and Pylyshyn 1981, p. 162.

18. Fodor and Pylyshyn 1981, p. 166.

representations contrasts with the idea that representational states are about non-nomic properties.[19] Given Fodor's overall position on representation, early vision should not count as representational because it does not comprise states that are about the distal environment.

According to the position outlined by Fodor and Pylyshyn themselves, then, we should be able to see percepts as produced by states that are not representations and misperception occurs precisely when the intermediaries are present—and cause the percept to occur—but the distal cause is not present. So it is not clear why Fodor and Pylyshyn insist on the need to understand vision inferentially. Misperceiving is not a reason to prefer inferentialism. It is only a reason to favor conceiving of percepts as states that can be accurate or inaccurate, and that are produced through the use of some causal intermediaries.

This completes the job that I set out to do in this section, but I want to end it with a brief aside concerning visual content and its richness because the issue of content is nicely connected to the issue of misperception in Fodor and Pylyshyn's article. Those uninterested in whether the embedded view has any bearing on how rich perceptual content is, can skip ahead to the next section.

Brief aside on visual content

Fodor and Pylyshyn's primary target in the article just discussed is Gibson's idea that we directly perceive affordances. Affordances are roughly properties of objects that elicit action in an organism.[20] For example, the properties of being edible or walk-on-able or climbable are all affordances because they are properties of objects that suggest an action to be performed with (or on) the objects perceived. Such properties are important components of Gibson's story of how perception and action interact in ecological settings.

What is relevant about affordances in the present context is that they are complex properties. They are—as the literature on perceptual content would call them—'high-level' properties, to be distinguished from 'low–level' properties such as colors and shapes. Many agree that the latter types of properties

---

19. Fodor 1987b, Fodor and Pylyshyn 1981, p. 165. See also section 3.3.

20. There is a substantial literature on what affordances are—for instance, whether they are relational or dispositional properties—and I do not have space to summarize the literature here. See Chemero 2003, Heft 1989, Norman 1999, Scarantino 2003, Stoffregen 2003, Turvey 1992. What I am about to discuss is orthogonal to what particular theory of affordances one holds.

are represented in perception: they are what perception paradigmatically tells us about. Recent interest is on whether more complex, high–level properties are also part of perceptual content.[21] It is a matter of recent dispute, for example, whether the property of being a pine tree or the property of being a cause can be perceived, and a number of considerations, including whether vision is affected by expertise, are thought to have a bearing on this issue.

In their article, Fodor and Pylyshyn deny that affordances are perceived *directly*. They are properties that can only be represented after an inference. Thus edibility can only be represented as the result of first representing the appearance (color and shape) of an object. Misperception is one component of Fodor and Pylyshyn's argumentative strategy. If misperceiving requires the perceptual process to be an inference from sensory representations about the proximal world to percepts, then we have reason to suppose that high-level properties, such as affordances, are not perceived directly. Indeed they may not be perceived at all, depending on how we define the outputs of visual inferences.

If the considerations of this section are cogent, however, then this line of reasoning does not go through. Inferences are not required for misperceiving. We can misperceive edges or three-dimensional objects even if perception is direct and embedded. So accepting EV has consequences for whether affordances can be perceived directly, and for the more general question of the richness of perceptual content.

In the embedded account, an object or item in space is perceived directly because—presuming that it is useful for us to perceive it—the object is fairly frequent in our environment, and there is a significant statistical correlation between *it* and the type of stimulation that it reflects on the retina. The fact that this correlation is probabilistic is one of the things that explains occasional error. It follows that the question of whether affordances are perceived directly can be addressed by looking at whether they are relatively ubiquitous in our environment, and at whether there is a significant statistical correlation between *them* and the stimuli that are projected on the retina when they are present. This is ultimately an empirical question to be answered with the tools of Natural Scene Statistics.

If we found that the properties of being edible or walk-on-able were statistically correlated to certain intensities of light, in a similar fashion to how, say, edges are statistically correlated with light discontinuities of a certain

21. Siegel 2006, 2009.

orientation, then we would have *some* reason to suppose that edibility and walk-on-ability are perceived directly. We can easily think of how perceiving affordances of this kind would be evolutionarily advantageous, and we seem to have plenty of behavioral evidence that our performance is sometimes stirred by the fact that something is edible and/or walk-on-able.

Vice versa, if edibility varied so much from object to object that things that are edible did not have any visible characteristics in common—that is, they did not project on the retina patterns of stimulation that are characteristic of edibility—we would have little reason to suppose that we perceive this type of affordance. Along similar lines, the question of whether we perceive other 'high–level properties,' such as the property of being a pine tree can be addressed by seeing if we find a statistically significant correspondence between the property in question and a certain pattern of retinal stimulation.

With this, I am not arguing for the claim that high-level properties are represented in perception. I am arguing that a way to find out whether they are is by looking at their utility, and at whether they produce characteristic patterns of stimulation. The embedded view offers a way of addressing issues of perceptual content that is independent of both the phenomenology of vision, and the question of whether perception is cognitively penetrable. The method that comes with the embedded view need not contrast with a phenomenological or knowledge-based method, and it might need to be integrated with them. Nevertheless, by reflecting on EV, we can outline an additional approach to address questions of content.

I conclude that misperception is not a problem for EV, and that it brings out a new angle from which to think of the richness of perception. Because vision is not inferential we can appreciate how a number of high-level properties may not only be seen, but seen directly.

4.5 Visual illusion

Like misperception, visual illusions involve a perceptual error where the world appears as it is not. Unlike misperceptions, however, illusions seem better fit to show that representational mediation is required in vision. This is because, in some illusions, the percept seems to be generated *via* a prior state that is also in error.

Illusions are often produced by artificial stimuli and there are many examples of them, so much so that a thorough survey would require another book. For simplicity, we can concentrate on one of the most popular and well-studied cases: the Müller-Lyer. This is an illusion involving size (see figure 4.1).

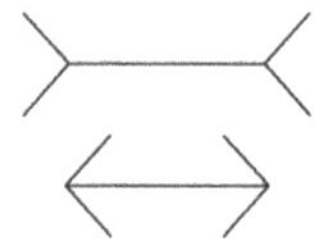

FIGURE 4.1 Müller-Lyer illusion. From Howe and Purves 2005a, p. 1235.

Despite knowledge that the two lines in the figure are equal in length, the top line (ending with the arrowtails) is typically seen as longer than the bottom line (ending with the arrowheads). One explanation of the illusion appeals to the fact that the lines are first (mis)represented as being at different distances from the observer.

In this section, I show that EV can adequately account for this sort of illusion. I first look at two important cognitive theories: the 'perspective theory' championed by Richard Gregory[22] and the 'incorrect comparison theory' proposed (among others) by Irvin Rock.[23] Neither theory withstands scrutiny. The perspective theory is ultimately inadequate, and the incorrect comparison theory is both compatible with EV and not as explanatory powerful as views based on Natural Scene Statistics.

Let's start by looking at the perspective theory. According to the perspective theory, the assumption of size constancy is implicated in producing the illusory percept in figure 4.1.[24] The basic idea is that the visual system represents the lines as located at different distances from the observer. This is because the arrowheads give depth cues that make the lines appear that way. You may notice, for instance, that the arrowheads make the lines look a bit like two edges. You may see them as the inside edge of a box further away from the observer, and as the outside edge of a box closer to the observer. Derivatively, the lines are represented as non-co-planar and this is a misrepresentation of the lines since, in reality, they lie on the same plane.[25]

Because the lines are represented as being at different distances, the assumption of size constancy kicks in. This assumption—recall from section 4.3—is the assumption that entities in the world retain their size despite changes, due to distance, in the dimensions of their retinal projection. By using constancy, the visual system adjusts the size of objects perceived

22. Gregory 1963.

23. Rock 1997, ch. 22.

24. Fodor 1984, p. 33, Gregory 1963.

25. If the lines do not look to you as differing in distance, then suppose that you represent the lines that way without being aware of it.

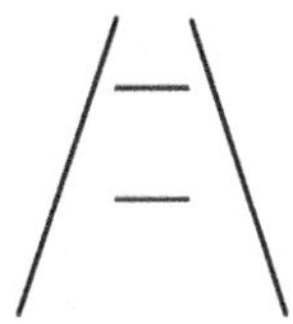

FIGURE 4.2 Ponzo illusion. From Fineman and Carlson 1973, p. 32.

to be further away, typically producing accurate representations. If an object moves further away, for example, it will be enlarged a bit.

This gives us an illuminating way of explaining the Müller-Lyer illusion. According to the perspective theory, the two lines in the illusion are represented as being at different distances. The visual system adjusts their size for size constancy and makes one appear bigger than the other. In particular, the system makes the one that appears to be further away look bigger.

A positive aspect of this theory is that it appears capable of explaining other illusions that seemingly involve depth cues, such as the Ponzo illusion (see figure 4.2). In this illusion, the two oblique lines are depth cues. They give the impression of receding in the distance (roughly, as train tracks would do in a natural environment). Accordingly, the top horizontal line is seen to be further away, and its size is correspondingly increased for size scaling. In the case of both illusions, the explanation requires that we think of vision as representationally mediated. The visual system first represents two objects at different distances, and then, given the assumption of size constancy, infers that one is bigger than the other, representing them to be that way.

Direct accounts, by contrast, seem particularly inept at explaining how the illusions are produced. Since the lines are the same length, their retinal projection is also the same. If what we perceive were a direct result of the visual stimulus, we should perceive the lines to be equal. We do not, however. In explaining why we do not, appeal to simple causal and functional intermediaries is not helpful. What is relevant of such intermediaries, in these cases, is that they stand for something that is both absent and distal. The intermediaries stand for lines at different distances, and they should count as representations.

If this were right it would be an instructive result. As I have been keen to point out, whether representations are needed to explain certain kinds of visual phenomena is an open empirical question.

As it turns out, however, the perspective theory proves to be an inadequate account of the 'depth illusions.' This is primarily because depth cues, and representing the lines to be at different distances are not necessary—and

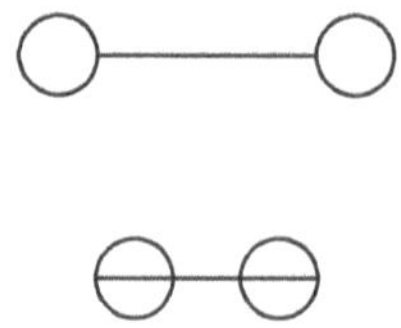

FIGURE 4.3 Müller-Lyer figure with no depth cues. From Purves and Lotto 2011, p. 121.

are likely not involved at all—in perceiving the lines as differing in length. A convergence of empirical results demonstrates that this is the case.

It was first noted that the illusory percept is generated by figures that contain no depth cues such as figure 4.3.[26] If the illusion were caused by taking the lines to be non-co-planar, then removal of depth cues should alter the illusion. Presumably, the no-depth display should affect the representation of distance. But this is not the case. The illusion occurs more or less unaltered in figure 4.3.

Additionally, the perspective theory predicts that the illusory perception should be enhanced when we add depth cues that are consistent with the ones given by the arrowheads. *Vice versa* the illusion should decrease when the added depth cues contrast with the cues given by the arrowheads. This is because if depth played a causal role in generating the illusion, then enhancing depth should also enhance the strength of the illusion. This, however, is not the case. Increasing or decreasing depth cues does not correspondingly alter the illusion. This is true of both the Müller-Lyer and the Ponzo figures.[27]

Three more pieces of evidence are puzzling given the perspective theory: one is that pigeons, animals that have trouble perceiving depth in two-dimensional drawings, are found to be sensitive to both the Müller-Lyer and the Ponzo illusions.[28] The other is that the illusory percepts occur also in the presence of three–dimensional shapes that resemble the two-dimensional drawing, where the shapes do not appear to be at different distances.[29] Finally, detaching the brackets from the horizontal lines is found to reverse the illusion: the line with the arrowheads (< >) appears longer than the one with the

26. Ahluwalia 1978, Howe and Purves 2005a, 2005b.

27. Fujita 1997, Hamaguchi 2001.

28. Fujita 2001, Fujita et al. 1991, Nakamura et al. 2006.

29. Rock 1997, ch. 20.

arrowtails (><), a fact that is not predicted by the theory.[30] This converging evidence indicates that representing the lines to be at different distances is not necessary, and that depth cues are not needed.

What other explanation is available? An alternative theory is the 'incorrect comparison theory.'[31] I discuss it here because, for reasons that are somewhat opaque to me, this theory is sometimes seen as just a version of the perspective theory.

According to the incorrect comparison theory, what is crucial to explain the illusions is not the representation of depth, but rather the representation of the lines as belonging to a three-dimensional object.[32] I noted earlier that the arrowheads make the lines look like two edges, and this may suggest that what is centrally involved in perceiving the illusion are not distance and size constancy, but the capacity to represent the two-dimensional drawing in three dimensions. The idea is that the horizontal lines are seen to be different in size because they form part of a bigger and a smaller object. So perceiving the illusion presupposes being able to see objects in three dimensions.

This account of the Müller-Lyer illusion is supported by a number of empirical facts. The illusion is found to be reduced when the brackets attached to the horizontal lines are a different color than the lines.[33] This reduction is predicted by the fact that, in this scenario, the lines and the brackets may not be represented as belonging to the same object.

The occurrence and magnitude of the illusion is also affected by whether the illusory display is seen monocularly or binocularly, with the latter increasing the illusory effect.[34] Since binocular vision is also involved in perceiving objects in three dimensions, this is further suggestive of the plausibility of the incorrect comparison theory.

The illusion is additionally impaired in patients with damaged superior (and inferior) parietal cortex. These brain areas are usually involved in three dimensional object perception.[35]

Although some of its proponents take the incorrect comparison theory to be a version of the perspective theory in demonstrating the indirect nature

30. Nakamura et al. 2006, Yanagisawa 1939.

31. Matlin and Foley 1997, Rock 1997, ch. 20.

32. Nanay 2009, p. 579.

33. Coren and Girgus 1972.

34. Papert 1961.

35. Nanay 2009, Weidner and Fink 2007.

of vision,[36] it is hard to see why this is the case. Admitting that the ability to see three-dimensional objects is presupposed in seeing the 'depth illusions' does not amount to conceding that vision is representationally mediated. It is not that, like in the perspective-theory-style of explanation, we need to first represent the lines as belonging to a three dimensional object of a certain size, and then infer that the lines are different in size. It is rather that, as we see that the lines belong to 3*D* objects that have different sizes, we also see them as differing in size. Since—with the embedded view—we have a story of how we get representations of three-dimensional objects that have certain sizes without inferences, EV seems perfectly compatible with the incorrect comparison theory. According to such a theory, we see the lines as different simply because we see them as belonging to different-sized objects.

But in fact arguing for this compatibility is not necessary as there is a plausible alternative model that explains the Müller-Lyer, as well as other depth illusions, without appeal to either the representation of depth or to the ability to represent objects in three dimensions. This model comes, again, from Natural Scene Statistics.

Notice, first, that not all aspects of the evidence reported previously are accounted for by the incorrect comparison theory. The results on pigeons, for instance, are puzzling given their proven inability to see three-dimensional shapes in two-dimensional figures. Further, it is a notable and problematic fact of the Müller-Lyer that neither the brackets nor the horizontal lines are needed to elicit a misperception of the spatial interval.[37] Figures 4.4 and 4.5 demonstrate this fact.

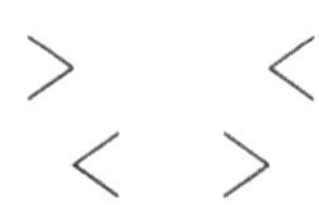

FIGURE 4.4 Müller-Lyer figure with no lines. From Howe and Purves 2005a, p. 1235.

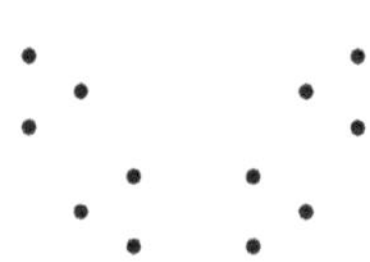

FIGURE 4.5 Müller-Lyer figure with no brackets. From Howe and Purves 2005a, p. 1235.

36. Rock 1997, p. 314.

37. Howe and Purves 2005a, p. 1234.

Given the absence of cues that signal the presence of three-dimensional objects, the incorrect comparison theory seems to have a hard time predicting the illusory effects in figures 4.4 and 4.5. These effects are predicted by an alternative model that looks at the statistical relationship between image and environmental source.

In the Müller-Lyer case, the lines or intervals appear to be different in length because the stimulus that they, together with the brackets, produce is likely caused by environmental sources that differ in length. This was found by sampling a large number (about 10^6) of images of natural scenes, some containing few if any human artifacts, and some depicting man-made environments. The images were analyzed for sets of pixels whose positions matched the geometrical configuration of the Müller-Lyer. Researchers started by identifying, say, one of the brackets of the illusion—such as an arrowtail—and then they looked for the presence, in the image, of the other components. If the other components were present, they deemed the image as containing the environmentally valid sources of the Müller-Lyer illusion.[38]

It was found that, in natural environments, if we start with the physical sources of the arrowtail, the other bracket is more likely to occur farther away than it would if the starting point had been the physical source of the arrowhead. This provides a neat explanation of the illusion. We see the lines as different in length because they project on the retina a stimulus that, in our environment, is likely caused by things that differ in length or in distance from each other. This is found to be true even for the variants of the illusion in figures 4.3, 4.4, and 4.5. And, as it turns out, this type of explanation can be applied to also explain other illusions not all of which involve three dimensionality or depth, such as the Poggendorff, Chubb, and Cornsweet illusions.[39]

This result is unsurprising in an embedded framework. The visual apparatus is sensitive to the stimulus projected on the retina and it is wired to process the stimulus in a way that reflects its past successes. Given the retinal projection of the illusion, the system produces representations of lines differing in length because, in our world, that stimulus is more often than not caused by elements differing in length. In other words, the system processes the stimulus in the way that it was (and it is) wired to do to probably get things right (or to probably get what is advantageous to get).

---

38. Howe and Purves 2005a, pp. 1234–1235.

39. Howe et al. 2005, Long and Purves 2003, Lotto and Purves 2001, Lotto et al. 1999, Purves et al. 1999.

Forming illusory percepts directly is then far from a mystery. It is just what we should expect given statistical regularities and the normal causes of the stimuli present in illusory displays. The further attempt of visual systems to reduce error—in the spirit of predictive coding—accounts for diachronic changes in illusory percepts. Prolonged exposure to illusions may change their appearance because the visual system engages in a continuous effort to adjust to the stimulus. But if this is true, then an embedded understanding of visual processing is in a position to explain visual illusions and their appearance over time.

4.6 Completion

Perceptual completion, sometimes referred to as perceptual 'filling in,' is the phenomenon that occurs when subjects report perceiving something in a particular region that is absent from that region, but suggested by contextual factors. There are many different kinds of completion.[40] For reasons of simplicity, we can concentrate on figure 4.6.

Observers report seeing a complete circle covered by a square. This is despite the fact that only a 'pac-man' portion of the circle is visible. Perceiving objects or figures as complete when they are not entirely visible is called 'amodal completion.' The objects are perceived as complete even if observers do not *see* all parts of them: they are perceived, despite not being perceived in any particular modality.[41]

Amodal completion is a ubiquitous occurrence in natural environments, where objects are never in full view—that is, we always have only a perspective on them. Evidence for it is fairly robust.[42] Groups of neurons in the visual

FIGURE 4.6 Occluded circle.

40. Pessoa et al. 1998.

41. Kanizsa and Gerbino 1982.

42. The evidence answers skeptical worries raised with regard to completion. Daniel Dennett argues that, despite appearances, perceptual experience is strikingly *dis*continuous. The brain is not in the business of filling in or giving detail, but in the business of finding out (Dennett 1992, p. 47). *Contra* Dennett, the studies reported here, offer fairly convincing and non-subjective support for the idea that completion occurs and is a genuine perceptual phenomenon.

cortex of monkeys are sensitive to complete objects and to partly occluded ones, but not to fragmented objects.[43] Completion is found in a number of non-linguistic non-human animals, such as squirrel monkeys, Japanese macaques, rhesus macaques, baboons, and chimpanzees (but, somewhat surprisingly, not in pigeons).[44] In humans, a number of psychophysical effects confirm that observers see occluded objects as complete: the afterimage of an occluded rectangle is found to consist of an image where the completed rectangle and its occluders alternate.[45] Moreover, as we saw in section 3.6, occluded figures have priming effects on judgments of similarity that are almost identical to the priming effects of complete figures.[46] Given this evidence, we need to explain how visual systems achieve completion.

A recent review of the literature suggests that different neurological mechanisms may be responsible for different instances of the phenomenon.[47] Quite apart from how completion may be realized at the neuronal level, however, a single theoretical framework can be offered to explain the process in its different occurrences.

The, by now familiar, inferential idea is to see completion as the solution to a problem.[48] The problem is that of reconstructing the layout of a scene despite the poverty of the stimulation coming from it, due to occlusion and cluttering. The brain—in particular the visual system—is said to solve this problem by *interpreting* the fragmented visual input in terms of completed objects, where this interpretation is again understood as a representationally mediated inference. The brain is said to deploy internal resources—p- and s-representations—that *add information* to what is available to the eye, and this explains why we often perceive more than what is present.[49]

---

43. Sugita 1999, Grosof et al. 1993.

44. Bakin et al. 2000, Deruelle et al. 2000, Fagot et al. 2006, Fujita 2001, Nagasaka and Osada 2000, Nagasaka and Wasserman 2008, Sato et al. 1997, Sekuler et al. 1996, Sugita 1999, Ushitani and Fujita 2005.

45. Bozzi 1980.

46. Sekuler and Palmer 1992.

47. Pessoa et al. 1998.

48. Rock and Anson 1979.

49. See Palmer 1999 and Sekuler and Palmer 1992. Stephen Palmer writes:

> Perhaps the clearest and most convincing evidence that visual perception involves the construction of environmental models comes from the fact that our perceptions include portions of surfaces that we cannot actually see.
>
> (Palmer 1999, p. 10)

In bottom-up inferential views, the visual system represents the presence of fragments in the scene and then interprets the fragments as complete objects based on some stored knowledge of the world. In explaining the way we perceive figure 4.6, for example, we suppose that the visual system first represents the pac-man shape and then infers the presence of a full circle by assuming that pac-man shapes adjacent to a figure are typically circles covered by the figure.

In top-down constructive views, the system may start off preferring hypotheses that concern complete objects, thereby employing a prior or hyper-prior that assigns higher probability to hypotheses about complete entities. The system then checks the hypothesis against the sensory evidence. Since pac-man shapes are typically occluded circles the initial hypothesis is confirmed. In both types of accounts, sensory representations of the pac-man, and representations of principles—for instance, that if a pac-man adjacent to a figure is present then a complete circle is present—are employed in processing.

This kind of inferential explanation transfers well to everyday situations where completion is ubiquitous. We perceive objects in the environment as complete even if only parts of them are visible. We tend to perceive objects as, for instance, rigid and three dimensional, even if we are exposed only to their surfaces. It is as if the visual system implicitly *knew* what objects in the environment are typically like and produced representations of them given such knowledge.

By contrast, completion seems mysterious in direct paradigms. If the stimulus for vision wholly determined what we see, then, since the stimulus is fragmented, our visual world should also be fragmented. That this is not the case stands against direct accounts.

He adds:

> Completion presents an even more compelling case for the constructive view of visual perception than do illusions and ambiguous figures. It shows that what you perceive actually goes a good deal beyond what is directly available in the light reaching your eyes. You have very strong expectations about what self-occluded and partly occluded surfaces are like. There must be construal from something more than the light entering your eyes, because the image itself contains no direct stimulation corresponding to these perceived, but unseen, parts of the world.
>
> (Palmer 1999, p. 11)

If the idea behind the embedded view is clear enough, however, then we can explain completion in an embedded framework without appeal to representational intermediaries. To introduce why this is the case, notice, again, that EV does not deny that visual operations involve a process that may happen in stages, that takes time, and that is biased in some way. What EV denies is that this process consists in an inference.

Take the general problem of understanding how the visual system moves from informationally poor to informationally rich or useful states. The embedded view presumes that the visual system relies on facts about the world to produce what is informationally rich from what is informationally impoverished. The system detects edges when tracking light discontinuities because of the fact that light discontinuities are caused by edges. In a sense, the environment in which the visual system is situated *adds information* to the one contained in the initial states. The environment shaped, and continues to shape, the visual apparatus to develop direct connections between states that track discontinuities and states that track edges. No additional representational complexity is in place.

Along the same lines, the embedded view explains completion. By tracking contextual factors (like pac-man shapes) the visual system relies on the environment to produce representations. In our world, circular fragments adjacent to a figure are often complete and covered circles. The visual apparatus does not need to encode this fact. It is simply wired to conform to it because complete (covered) circles are the typical causes of the stimulus configuration. One type of neuronal pattern that picks up on fragments simply activates another. So completion is achieved without an inferential process.[50]

To suppose, like inferentialists do, that the intermediaries of completion are representations we would need additional evidence and we lack such evidence. Take, first, the suggestion that visual perception employs intermediate sensory representations. We saw in section 3.6 that, despite attempts to prove otherwise, we lack evidence for this view. The study testing the priming effects of completion shows that we have little reason to suppose that the representation of a complete figure is preceded by a representation of the visible fragments of the figure.

---

50. This explanation of how completion is achieved does not make reference to action, thereby differing from enactive explanations of the phenomenon (Noë 2002). It is worth noting, however, that enactive approaches are geared at explaining not just (or not even primarily) the ontogenesis of completion (like EV does) but (also) its phenomenology. As far as I can tell, enactive accounts of completion are compatible with the embedded view.

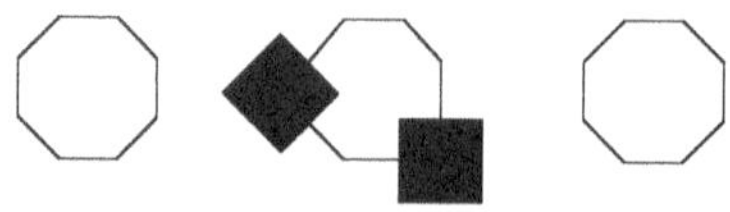

FIGURE 4.7 Occluded octagon. From Kanizsa 1985, p. 30.

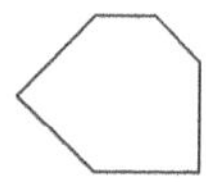

FIGURE 4.8 Un-occluded irregular figure. From Kanizsa 1985, p. 31.

Consider, next, the idea that completion presupposes the representation of some assumptions about the world that serve to add information to the one contained in the sensory states. Non-cognitivists about completion often notice that the process happens in early vision, and that it is plausibly associative, since it is *insensitive* to contrary information.[51]

In a number of studies, Gaetano Kanizsa and his collaborators show that occluded figures are often completed in a way that seems odd within the 'logic' of the context. Given the nearby flankers, it would make sense for the occluded geometrical figure represented in Figure 4.7 to be completed as an octagon, but this is not the case. Figure 4.8 is a better representation of how the figure is completed by the visual system. Indeed the appearance of the figure is not (easily) changed by paying attention to the suggestive surrounding figures.

Taking this fact into consideration, Kanizsa writes:

> The conclusion that can be drawn from these demonstrations is that the visual system, in the cases in which it is free to do so, does not always choose the solution that is most coherent with the context, as normal reasoning would require. This means that seeing follows a different logic—or, still better, that it does not perform *any reasoning at all* but simply works according to autonomous principles of organization which are not the same principles which regulate thinking.
>
> (Kanizsa 1985, pp. 32–33 [emphasis added])

The insensitivity to 'logic' of the visual process in completion is a suggestive result. It does not *imply* that the visual system is not rule-following,

51. Kanizsa 1985, p. 28, Kanizsa and Gerbino 1982.

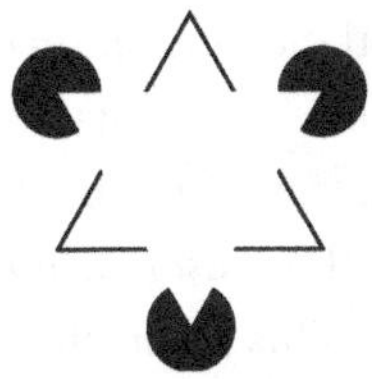

FIGURE 4.9 Kanizsa triangle. Sterman 1994.

since something can perform inferences while being widely irrational.[52] Yet the result raises the question of what other reasons one has for supposing that vision is inferential. Insensitivity to logic indicates that the idea of a wired visual system is a standing hypothesis, a hypothesis that is capable of explaining how completion is achieved without appeal to a representationally mediated process.

Now, in closing this section, I want to remark that despite the various successes of EV outlined in this section and chapter, the embedded hypothesis is an *empirical* hypothesis. There may be cases where introducing a representationally mediated process is necessary. I regard this as a positive, rather than a negative feature of the embedded view since standing hypotheses concerning visual processing should be testable and open to counter examples. To illustrate this point, consider the fairly famous Kanizsa triangle (figure 4.9).

Two types of completion, modal and amodal, occur in this figure. Observers report seeing a bright white triangle with relatively clear boundaries, superimposed on three black circles and a second triangle. Both the boundaries and the brightness change of the foreground triangle are illusory. There is no corresponding luminance difference between the triangle and the ground. This is called 'modal completion': what observers report seeing is not present in the scene and has properties, such as brightness, that are typical of the visual modality.[53]

In addition, observes report seeing the illusory triangle as covering three complete black circles and a second triangle. This is despite the fact that only portions of the circles and of the triangle are visible. As we saw, perceiving objects as complete even when they are not entirely visible because parts of them are covered or occluded is called 'amodal completion.'

We have reason to suppose that EV has a hard time explaining the perception of this figure. This is because the perception of the circles as complete

52. More on this issue in section 4.8.

53. Michotte et al. 1964.

and covered seems to depend on the perception of an illusory triangle—that is, it seems to depend on a representational state that stands for something not present and distal. In simple cases of completion—such as figure 4.6—the embedded visual system tracks the presence of fragments and is wired to process them as complete entities. This same story is not applicable in this new case. If the perception of the covered circles depends on the perception of the illusory triangle, then the transition between these two states is a transition between representations. In the absence of an alternative explanation—for example, an explanation in terms of Natural Scene Statistics—the Kanizsa triangle seems explicable only by supposing that vision is representationally mediated.

This result is, perhaps, due to the artificial nature of the stimulus. We may appeal, here, to Gibson's repeated remarks that the tendency to understand vision as involving representations is due to testing it in non-natural and impoverished environments. In the natural world, complete objects are typically covered by real, non-illusory occluders, which can simply be tracked.

Regardless of whether this is right, we should accept the result as instructive, and as how it should be. Vision may be cognitive in some cases.[54] Yet this result also highlights that the need to appeal to representational intermediaries is at least exaggerated in contemporary cognitive psychology. In many paradigmatic cases, vision is non-cognitive.

The next two sections strengthen this point by showing that the embedded view is also compatible with, and capable of explaining, instances of visual flexibility. These cases seem to be particularly problematic for accounts that view the visual system as wired.

In what follows, I provide an embedded way of understanding multi-stability, showing that seeing the same figure or object in multiple ways does not require an inferential process. I then conclude the chapter by discussing cases of cognitive penetrability, and showing that they also do not constitute a problem for EV.

4.7 Multi-stability

We normally see the world in a stable way: we tend to see the objects around us in pretty much the same way through time. Bearing some differences in

54. Although it may still not be inferential in any substantive sense. Admitting that vision is mediated by representations does not amount to admitting that it is mediated by represented assumptions.

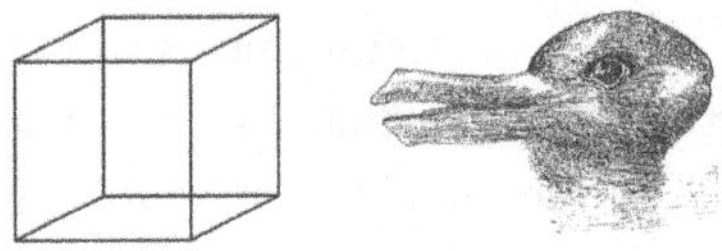

FIGURE 4.10 Bi-stable Necker cube (left); duck-rabbit (right). Right image from Jastrow 1899.

illumination and position, things appear to maintain their shape, color, orientation, and many of their other properties in a way that is hard (and sometimes contingently impossible) to change. Our perceptual world is remarkably stable, and how we see it seems to often escape our control. Indeed, in the case of visual illusions, it is stable against our own best judgment. We see the illusory percept in pretty much the same way even after we learn that it is illusory.

There are, however, cases in which this stability fails. Ambiguous figures are a particularly good example of this failure (see figure 4.10).

Images like the ones in figure 4.10 can be seen in two (and sometimes more) mutually exclusive ways, suggesting that perception can be quite flexible. In some instances, we can shift from seeing one thing to another and we have some measure of command over the shifts, switching from one percept to the other at will.[55]

Experiencing multiple percepts is not limited to ambiguous figures. Despite their usual stability, ordinary objects can also be seen in new ways. If observed for a period of time, a dark doorknob may appear to be a concave hole, a trashcan may look like a small stool, and a crack in the wall may look like a crawling bug. In such cases, as in the case of the images in figure 4.10, the same stimulus may give rise to two or more distinct percepts.

The fact that, in these cases, we have some command over what we see may suggest that multi-stability is a phenomenon at the intersection of seeing and thinking.[56] Like in imagining, we have some power over what we see. Yet because shifts also depend quite heavily on the stimulus, they are typically considered to be within the purview of perceptual theory. We *see* the image or the object in one way or another; we don't just *imagine* the images or objects to be that way.

Shifts are paradigmatic visual cases that, like illusions, occur in nonhuman animals such as pigeons.[57] A good account of vision must explain how

55. Churchland 1989.

56. Budd 1987, Wittgenstein 1953.

57. Vetter et al. 2000.

they are possible. Preferably, a satisfactory theory would also explain the characteristics of switching mentioned earlier. In some instances, no matter how hard we try, we are unable to see an object or figure any differently from how we typically do. In these cases we are heavily constrained in what we see. In other cases we seem to have some jurisdiction over how we see an item, and we may be able to perceive it in a new and unexpected way.

Once again, inferential accounts seem to be in a better position than direct accounts to explain multi-stability because they conceive of vision as involving an interpretation where encoded knowledge is used to derive different percepts. Stephen Palmer says:

> Ambiguous figures demonstrate the constructive nature of perception because they show that perceivers interpret visual stimulation and that more than one interpretation is sometimes possible. If perception were completely determined by the light stimulating the eye, there would be no ambiguous figures because each pattern of stimulation would map onto a unique percept. This position is obviously incorrect. Something more complex and creative is occurring in vision, going beyond the information strictly given in the light that stimulates our eyes.
>
> (Palmer 1999, p. 10)

Proponents of Bayesian models voice a similar sentiment:

> The fact that the very same figure can be interpreted in two different ways with a mere rotation indicates that the visual system is using additional knowledge beyond the stimulus information.
>
> (Mamassian et al. 2002, p. 23)

It is somewhat curious that, in cognitive accounts, appeal to inferences serves to explain both why vision is stable in the face of underdetermined retinal stimuli, and why it is *not* stable in the presence of ambiguous figures. One might think that we would need some additional explanation for why stability is violated in certain cases (more on this later).

An interpretive process seems necessary, however, because an ambiguous figure projects on our retinas a single pattern of stimulation. If vision were direct we should see a single thing. The fact that we do not indicates that something more is involved in reconstructing the percept, and this invites the thought that an interpretation is involved.

We can, however, preserve this intuition while pointing out that an interpretation is not necessarily an inference that requires representational structures. As we saw in the present chapter and throughout the book, inferentialists often use the terms 'inference,' 'construction,' and 'interpretation' interchangeably. Following this practice, I also used these terms interchangeably. Yet the identification between inferring, interpreting, and constructing is not mandatory, and the fact that it is not comes out nicely in multi-stability.

While it is natural to talk of an ambiguous figure or object as being interpreted in various ways, it is not clear that, when we talk this way, we intend to describe an inferential process. Unlike in other visual cases, it is far from straightforward how the idea of an inference would help.

That an inference is involved in multi-stability supposedly means that different encoded assumptions or principles can be used in processing the stimulus. In our usual and simplified example, light discontinuities at the retina may be caused by edges, lines, shadows, and many other environmental conditions. The visual apparatus might sometimes assume that a discontinuity in light intensity is caused by an edge and sometimes assume that it is caused by a shadow, thus producing different perceptions of the same environmental entity.

It is a bit harder to see what the assumptions should be in cases like the Necker cube or the duck-rabbit in figure 4.10. Vision scientists typically talk about assumptions concerning edges, surfaces, rigidity, convexity, and size, and some of these can perhaps help with the Necker cube. But they can hardly be the whole story of how we can see, say, a figure first as duck-shaped and then as rabbit-shaped.

Perhaps we need to ascribe to visual systems not only encoded principles concerning edges and surfaces, but also assumptions concerning ducks and rabbits. This would be somewhat implausible given that the assumptions are supposed to be proprietary to vision, but the crucial point is that we do not need to do it. For, it seems that an embedded framework can explain multistability without appeal to encoded instructions. This is because we can think of whatever assumptions vision needs, not as represented within it, but as describing how the visual apparatus is biased to function.

Just like vision can make use of different encoded rules, it can also rely on different environmental facts, where this means that, as a result of environmental pressure, it has functional features that make it process the same stimulus differently over time. When presented with a discontinuity in light intensity, the visual system can, in some cases, be wired to process it as an edge (because edges are the typical causes of the given discontinuity) and, in some cases, be wired to process it as a shadow (because shadows sporadically cause that same discontinuity). Similarly, we can imagine the visual system representing the presence of something duck-shaped or of something rabbit-shaped when doing so accords with the retinal stimulus. The system does not interpret the stimulus as produced by something rabbit-shaped in the sense of performing an *inference*. It rather interprets it in the sense of being wired by the fact that a given retinal projection may be typically (or often) caused by something that looks like a rabbit.[58]

Admittedly, this preliminary explanation of embedded multi-stable perception leaves much to be desired. One thing that is unexplained is why the shifts happen at all. It is unclear why the visual system would, given the same stimulation, sometimes rely on different facts to produce different percepts. We need to explain what conditions prompt the shifts given that perception is typically stable.

Notice, however, that this is a problem for *everybody* in the present dialectical context. Even those who accept a cognitive or inferential account need to explain why shifts happen. Appealing to an inference, on top of being problematic—because it is not clear how it helps—is also not sufficient to account for why we sometimes get two percepts rather than the usual one by looking at a single object or figure. We still need an explanation why the visual system sometimes uses different assumptions to process the same stimulation.

Reflecting on binocular rivalry suggests a first solution to this problem. Recall, from section 2.4, that in rivalry the eyes are isolated and exposed each to different stimuli—for instance, to the images of a face and a house. This exposure is plausibly responsible for the shift from one percept to the other because the total stimulus is clearly ambiguous and suggestive of different causes. The pattern of light that hits the eyes, in this case, is highly unstable.

In typical cases of multi-stability, we have both eyes exposed to the same image, but we can also think of the stimulus as ambiguous by appealing to its statistical properties. The idea is that certain light patterns, although in principle compatible with an infinity of distal conditions, have, in our environment, one or two (or a few more) typical causes. Unlike stable stimuli, that have only one typical cause, some patterns have more than one. They are as likely to be caused by, say, an edge as they are to be caused by shadows (and

58. Indeed we could build wired systems such as smoke detectors to do multi-stable signaling by taking advantage of the fact that smoke is an ambiguous input, being generated by both fire and other causes such as running cars. See Orlandi 2012a for this example.

we assume that both are pretty important for organisms like us to detect). If we follow the discussion of brightness constancy in section 4.3 we can give a sense of this ambiguity by thinking that some discontinuities in light intensity are blurry in a duplicitous way. They are not quite fuzzy enough to be shadows, but they are also not sharp enough to be uncontroversially edges. Discontinuities in light intensity of this kind are not just ambiguous in principle but ambiguous *in practice*. In our environment, they are as likely caused by edges as they are by shadows. It would then be *un*surprising if such discontinuities were implicated in bi-stable perception.

Similarly, some stimuli may be as likely caused by something duck-shaped, as they are by something rabbit-shaped. When this is the case, perception is predictably unstable. Shifts, in these circumstances, are caused exogenously by the ambiguity of retinal projections. Given the ambiguity of the stimulus the visual apparatus is wired in such a way that it switches from signaling one thing to signaling the other. If we want to think of this in terms of predictive coding models, we can think of the visual system as wired to reduce error, and as switching from one high-level hypothesis to another in an attempt to accommodate the duplicitous input. In multi-stability both eyes are exposed to the same thing, but, as in binocular rivalry, the stimulus is ambiguous enough to produce different percepts.

In providing this explanation, we appeal *not* to internal representational structures but to external circumstances. Just like we did in the case of stability and constancy, we appeal to external environmental and statistical conditions that have biased the visual apparatus to function as it does. This accounts for why, no matter how hard we try, we may be unable to see an object or figure any differently from how we typically do. What we see is heavily constrained by the statistical properties of the stimulus. If the stimulus has, in our environment, only one typical cause, we will likely experience only one percept.

The first stage in explaining the instability of perception, then, consists in appealing to the contingent instability of perceptual stimulation. This is only part of the story of multi-stability, however. I think that it identifies an important step for being able to experience shifts. But switching can also be prompted *exogenously*, and this marks an important difference between general multi-stability and binocular rivalry. In some cases, a shift is not driven (solely) by the ambiguity of the stimulus: we can have a measure of control over switching and, although this is not easy to do, we can occasionally see things in novel ways even when, previously, we could not.

In order to explain this fact, we need to appeal to more than just a certain way of understanding visual processing. In the rest of this section, I want to focus, in particular, on the role of visual search and attention.[59]

There is a growing literature concerning what attention consists of, and the different kinds of attentional mechanisms that humans (and non-humans) are endowed with.[60] One thing that most theorists agree about is that the allocation of attention has a selective function. Attention selects, and enhances, the part of the stimulus that needs to be processed. It also filters out unwanted information—that is, it ignores conditions that are not to be processed, since they are not relevant to the production of behavior.[61]

Attention is found to have effects on the threshold at which a stimulus is detected, and to influence the attunement of physiological states to certain kinds of, particularly important, conditions.[62] The primary reason why attention has these functions is because of limited processing capacities on the part of biological organisms.

The characterization of attentional mechanisms as having a selective function appears to be true of focal attention, which is the ability used in tasks of object search and identification in cluttered environments. The direction of focal attention typically, but not invariably, coincides with the point of fixation, that is, the point where we foveate.[63] Focal attention, whether understood as a type of spotlight or as a type of cognitive unison,[64] is selective: when the task is identifying an object among others, it selects the stimulus to be processed and it ignores stimuli that are irrelevant.

If we think of observers as capable of directing focal attention not only to whole objects and figures but also to features of said objects and figures we can begin to see how visual multi-stability occurs endogenously. Given a stimulus that is contingently compatible with different distal causes—such as an ambiguous figure—focusing on some features of it, rather than on others, prompts the visual system to gradually process the stimulus given the features that are tracked initially. This delivers percepts that are determined both by

---

59. The idea of understanding shifts as driven by attentional focus is present in authors as different as Pylyshyn and Wollheim (Pylyshyn 1999, p. 358, Wollheim 1980, p. 222).

60. Mole 2011, Pylyshyn 2009.

61. Desimone and Duncan 1995, Goldstone 2003, Posner and Petersen 1990.

62. See section 4.8, Eberhardt et al. 2004, Goldstone 2003.

63. Posner and Petersen 1990.

64. Mole 2011.

what is initially tracked and by how the system is constrained or wired to process information. A different percept may be produced if one focuses on different initial features.

This partly explains the temporal dimension of multi-stable perception. One first sees a figure as duck-shaped and then as rabbit-shaped. The time taken to shift is plausibly used to perform visual exploration, where observers pay attention to different parts of a figure or object. Paying attention to some features exposes the visual apparatus to properties of the stimulus that are more likely associated with one environmental entity—such as something duck-shaped. Paying attention to others, by contrast, may uncover properties that are more likely associated with a different entity—such as something rabbit-shaped. In other words, certain elements of a figure may project on the retina a stimulus that is diagnostic of something duck-shaped. By paying attention to them, vision produces the corresponding representation. Other elements may, instead, be diagnostic of something rabbit-shaped favoring a shift when observers focus on them.

What emerges is a picture of switching where observers are out to find what is already present to the senses. Shifts can be prompted by curiosity and they do not involve an inference. This explains why we have a measure of control in multi-stability. Although this is not always true—as attentional mechanisms can also be controlled by exogenous factors[65]—we do have some command over focal attention and, consequently, over how we perceive the world.

Looking at the empirical evidence on the subject uncovers that this is a plausible way of understanding multi-stability. In adults, the part of a reversible figure that an observer focuses on has been shown to determine which percept the viewer experiences.[66] Neurological studies confirm the stimulation of frontal and parietal areas associated with the control of selective attention during reversals.[67] Further, patients with unilateral frontal brain damage have greater difficulty in shifting than do normal control subjects.[68]

Studies on ocular activity during reversals further support this picture. Shifting is a phenomenon that involves a number of ocular events. In particular, saccades prior to and during reversals are positively associated with the

65. Pylyshyn 2009, p. 3.

66. Chastain and Burnham 1975.

67. Britz et al. 2009, Kleinschmidt et al. 1998, Leopold and Logothetis 1999, Nakatani and van Leeuwen 2006, Sterzer and Kleinschmidt 2007, Tong et al. 2006.

68. Ricci and Blundo 1990.

process. They increase in the period leading to a shift, and in conditions where fixation instructions restrict them, the rate of switching is considerably reduced.[69] Since saccades are closely associated with shifts in spatial attention, this implicates attentional mechanisms in the switching process.[70]

The hypothesis that shifting is guided by attention is also able to account for a number of studies that purport to show the effects of knowledge on multi-stability. Knowledge that a figure or object is ambiguous and knowledge of the terms of the ambiguity are important elements of reversing.[71] Researchers found that, when subjects are informed that a figure is ambiguous, their chances of switching increase significantly.

This result is readily explained by the idea that multi-stability can be initiated by visual search. If subjects know that a figure can be seen in multiple ways, they are more likely to engage in visual exploration. Furthermore, by knowing the terms of the ambiguity, observers are more likely to guide attention to those features of the figure that are suggestive of one of the known interpretations. The results are unsurprising if we think of multi-stability as induced by attentional changes.

Research in other areas of psychology further supports this view: bilingual children at six years of age are more likely to experience reversals than their monolingual peers.[72] This result can be attributed to the fact that bilingual children develop control over selective attention earlier than monolingual children because they have to control two active language systems.[73]

Further, children younger than age 5 are usually unable to reverse ambiguous figures spontaneously. One proposed explanation of this fact is that children are unable to reverse because they lack a Theory of Mind—that is, they lack, among other things, the capacity to interpret. They do not understand that the same thing can be seen in different ways.[74] This proposal, however, runs at odds with research on autistic children. Autistic children, while famously impaired in Theory of Mind tasks, appear to have no trouble seeing ambiguous figures in different ways.[75] A more plausible way to

69. Glen 1940, Ito et al. 2003, Toppino 2003.

70. Orlandi 2012b, Slotnick and Yantis 2005.

71. Girgus et al. 1977, Rock and Mitchener 1992, Rock et al. 1994.

72. Bialystok and Shapero 2005.

73. Bialystok 2001, Bialystok and Martin 2004.

74. Gopnik and Rosati 2001.

75. Ropar et al. 2003.

explain children's inability to reverse is that frontal cortex, the brain area that likely controls selective attention, develops late in humans, reaching maturity only during adolescence.[76] The importance of frontal cortex for switching is confirmed by the fact that frequent and infrequent switchers differ in brain activation precisely in this area.[77]

If this is right, then we can given the beginning of a story of multi-stability in terms that are perfectly compatible with the embedded view. We do not need to appeal to an inference to make room for the possibility of shifting. Appeal to the statistical properties of the stimulus, and to attentional control accounts for both why perception is sometimes unstable, and for the characteristic features of multi-stability. The degree of ambiguity of the stimulus helps explain the degree to which vision is stable or unstable: if the stimulus is particularly ambiguous, it is likely to generate multiple percepts. *Vice versa*, a stable stimulus, is likely to correspond to a single percept. The capacity to direct and hold attention to different parts of a figure or object helps explain our measure of control over shifting. It explains why we are sometimes able to see old things in new ways.

More may need to be said to give a full explanation of multi-stable perception. It is an outstanding question, for example, whether seeing something as duck-shaped requires prior exposure to ducks or to duck shapes. Further, the type of seeing on display in multi-stability can be quite sophisticated. It is likely involved in the appreciation of works of art, and one may suppose that prior exposure to art and artifacts is required for this kind of mastery.

These outstanding questions, however, are questions for any account of visual processing. They are questions that plague any view, inferential or embedded. It is far from clear that they cannot be answered in a way that is compatible with EV. Expertise in a given domain, for example, is found to have measurable effects on the capacity to direct and hold attention.[78]

If this is true, the embedded view emerges as explanatorily and empirically sound. Contrary to widespread belief, we do not need to appeal to an inference, or to a representationally mediated process to make room for the possibility of multi-stability.

To summarize the chapter so far, I have shown that the embedded view is able to explain a number of paradigmatic visual phenomena, and that it is in fact more compatible with the empirical research that we have on those

76. Diamond 2002.

77. Nakatani and van Leuween 2006.

78. See section 4.8. Thanks to Charles Siewert for raising these issues.

phenomena. This is true for both cases where vision appears to be inflexible, as in stability, constancy, misperception, illusion, and completion, and for cases where it appears to be malleable, as in multi-stability. The impression that accounting for these cases requires appeal to an interpretation is fostered by a misunderstanding of the commitments of direct accounts of vision. Such accounts can appeal to functional intermediaries to do a good deal of explanatory work.

This completes the bulk of the task of showing that EV has sufficient explanatory power, but to conclude this chapter we should turn to one more puzzling visual case. The next section argues that the embedded view is also compatible with cognitive penetrability, or semantic effects on perception.[79]

4.8 Semantic effects and cognitive penetrability

While many aspects of vision seem to be impervious to influences from prior experience, there are many cases in which this isolation fails. What we know, believe, feel, and have experienced in the past seems to affect what we see in a way that suggests that vision is not wired. This section argues, to the contrary, that semantic effects are compatible with the visual system being embedded: they can be explained by appeal to attentional effects, and to the sensitivity of vision to contextual elements.

I start with a review of some purported cases of cognitive penetrability. These cases include instances where beliefs and expertise have effects on what we see. I point out that there is disagreement concerning whether all of the presented cases are *genuine* instances of cognitive penetrability, and this disagreement has consequences for the issue of the modularity of perception and for its epistemic status. I then focus on whether purported instances of penetrability show the visual system to be reason-responsive (and thus not wired). I argue for a negative answer. Regardless of whether the presented cases are genuine instances of semantic effects, they can all be explained in an embedded framework.

We can start with an intuition: experts in a given domain see the world differently from novices. For instance, the expert gardener sees many more varieties of trees than does the non-expert. To those familiar with a given

79. I use 'cognitive penetrability' and 'semantic effects' interchangeably. Both of these labels stand for the influence of other contentful/representational mental states on perception.

language (say Cyrillic) words on a page appear different compared to the way that they appear to non-speakers.[80]

This intuition is not a *mere* intuition. It is corroborated by a number of empirical results. Airplane mechanics identify, by looking, many more parts in a plane than do novices.[81] Expert gardeners distinguish and name more varieties of plants than do non-experts.[82] Skilled birdwatchers have greater discriminative abilities when it comes to classifying birds, and they are better at spotting them.[83] Master chess players can reconstruct a briefly presented chess configuration more accurately than beginners can.[84] Expert chick sexers are better and faster than novices at spotting male from female birds.[85] Finally, when experienced radiologists view chest X-ray images they are better able to spot and remember abnormalities than untrained observers are.[86]

Knowledge does not just affect recognitional and classificatory abilities. It is also thought to affect simple perceptual processes, such as color perception.[87] Knowing that something is a banana affects its appearance, making it look yellow even when it isn't. Similarly, knowledge of social categories affects the perception of brightness. Faces that are categorized as belonging to a black person are perceived as darker than equally light faces that are categorized as belonging to a white person.[88]

The far left face in figure 4.11 typically appears darker than the far right face even though the two faces are equally bright. Additionally, when exposed to an ambiguous face (middle two images) perception of brightness varies depending on the label: if the face is labeled 'black' it is seen as darker than if it is labeled 'white.'[89]

---

80. Siegel 2006, 2012, Siewert 1998.

81. Rosch et al. 1976.

82. Boster 1986.

83. Johnson and Mervis 1997.

84. de Groot 1965. This capacity is not attributable to better memory, as masters are not able to perform as well if the pieces are put randomly on the board. Underlying the masters' skill is likely their capacity to perceive the board in 'chunks' rather than piece by piece (Chase and Simon 1973).

85. Biederman and Shiffrar 1987.

86. Myles-Worsley et al. 1988.

87. Hansen et al. 2006.

88. Levin and Banaji 2006.

89. Levin and Banaji 2006. In the experiment observers had to adjust the luminance of a face given a reference face. Subjects consistently matched the faces with black features

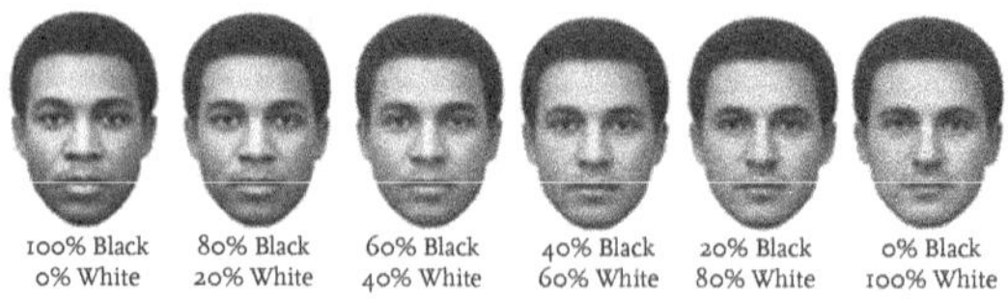

FIGURE 4.11 An equal-reflectance continuum between a black average face and a white average face. From Levin and Banaji 2006, p. 502.

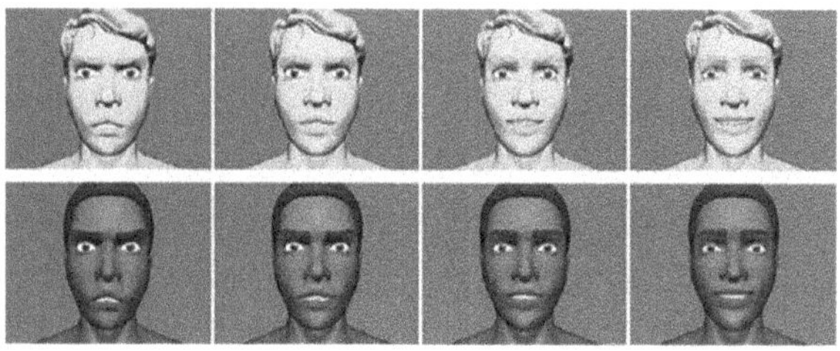

FIGURE 4.12 Four frames of an angry to happy movie. From Hugenberg and Bodenhausen 2003, p. 641.

In this example, perception of lightness seems to be sensitive to evidence. In particular, knowledge or assumptions about a given category seem to influence a basic visual function such as lightness perception. If one knows that a face belongs to a black person, then he will see it darker than it is.

Analogous effects occur when high-prejudiced white individuals look at ambiguous faces of white and black men. Such individuals judge black faces differently from the way they judge white faces.[90]

The black faces in figure 4.12, when presented sequentially as in a movie, are seen to transition from happiness to anger faster than the white faces with similar expressions. The prejudiced belief that black men tend to be more aggressive seems to affect face perception.

Effects of this kind are also found in less problematic contexts, such as the case of amodal completion.[91] In sections 3.7 and 4.6 I suggested that completion is often insensitive to 'logic,' since objects are often completed in a way that is odd given context. Indenting soft objects—such as a banana—are seen

---

with a less luminant sample. The 'label' result is complicated by the fact that observers may have adjusted the brightness of the face to reflect, not how they perceive it, but rather their knowledge primed by the label. We will, however, ignore this complication.

90. Hugenberg and Bodenhausen 2003.

91. Vrins et al. 2009. Thanks to Katalin Farkas for the reference.

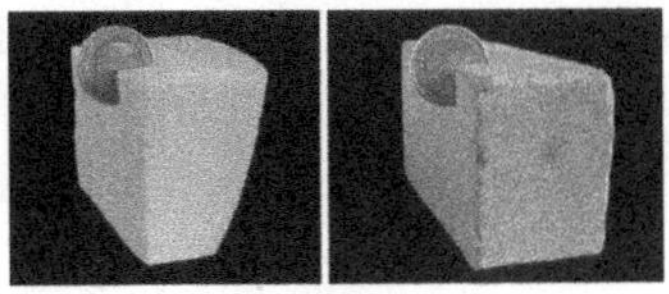

FIGURE 4.13 Two of the primes from Vrins et al. 2009, p. 20. Pion Ltd, London. S = soft; H = hard.

as complete and as penetrating other objects despite the fact that the item penetrated is much harder than they are—for instance, it is a brick of concrete. This insensitivity is not always the norm, however. While the consistency of the penetrating object does not make a difference to amodal completion, the hardness of the penetrated entity does. If a brick is visibly made of cheese or butter rather than of a hard material, subjects are more likely to complete the indenting elements.

When primed with a euro coin indenting a block of cheese (left image in figure 4.13) subjects are faster at judging that two complete circles are the same, while a similar effect is not found when the priming stimulus is the coin penetrating a concrete block (right image in figure 4.13). This suggests that observers tend to see the coin as complete only when the block is soft enough to allow indentation.[92]

In this case, amodal completion seems to vary systematically with what one knows about the surrounding context.

These perceptual effects are cases of what perceptual psychologists and philosophers call 'cognitive penetrability.' What one sees, rather than depending solely on stimulus conditions, also depends on one's background mental states. Beliefs concerning the color of one's skin, or the propensity of a certain social group toward anger have 'semantic effects' on perception, regardless of whether or not those beliefs are justified.

These are indeed only a small fraction of the studies that purport to show the effects of knowledge on perception, and a full survey is beyond the scope of this book. The proliferation of literature on this subject increased after a classic article published, in 1947, by Jerome Bruner and Cecile Goodman. In that article, Bruner and Goodman tried to present evidence that perception is affected by *emotive* states such as needing and valuing.

---

92. The results are a bit puzzling as this effect was only found for short exposition times to the prime (150 ms and 300 ms). For longer priming times (500 ms) exposure to the prime involving the hard brick significantly facilitated judgments of similarity between complete circles (Vrins et al. 2009, p. 27). We will ignore this complication, however.

The Bruner and Goodman study has since been discredited as there are problems with its setup and methodology, but the studies prompted a number of other attempts to show the influence of emotive states on perception.[93] Such attempts resulted in research that suggests that depression makes a difference to how one judges color,[94] and hunger may affect one's readiness to identify things as food.[95]

Historically, the issue of cognitive penetrability has been central to the debate concerning the modularity of perception. Proponents of modularity hold that perceptual processes, although inferential, are largely immune to influence from other mental faculties. Deniers, by contrast, claim that perception is informed by one's knowledge, expectations, and overall background theory.[96]

The debate concerning cognitive penetrability has also a bearing on the possibility of drawing a distinction between observation and theory.[97] Penetrability is thought to introduce epistemic problems for the neutrality of perception. If what we see is determined (in substantial part) by what we believe and want, then perception loses its status as an impartial and theory-independent tribunal. In particular, it is not clear how perception could serve to justify the beliefs that caused it, and how it could adjudicate between competing beliefs.[98]

93. In the Bruner and Goodman study, children were asked to adjust the size of a circle of light projected on a dark screen to match, first, the size of some presented coins varying from a penny through a half dollar and, then, the size of some gray cardboard discs. Children tended to overestimate the size of coins, suggesting that their valuing the coins affected their perception of size. Further, Bruner and Goodman compared the performance of well-off versus poor children on the same task, and found that the poor group overestimated the size of coins considerably more than did the rich group. One difficulty with the studies is that children were given the coins and discs to hold on the palm of their hands while making the comparison. This introduces tactual information as a possible complication for the results. The consistency of the different objects may have affected size perception. Additionally, the studies failed to replicate (Carter and Schooler 1949) and it was found that value has an effect on memory rather than on perception. It affects how big one *remembers* the coins to be.

94. Barrick et al. 2002.

95. Sanford 1936. See also Firestone and Scholl forthcoming, Stokes 2012, for a discussion of some more recent results.

96. See Fodor 1983 for a defense of modularity and Churchland 1979 for an anti-modular view.

97. Kuhn [1962]2012.

98. For recent discussion of some of these epistemological issues see Lyons 2011, Siegel 2012.

Central to these debates is whether the reported effects are effects on perception or on perceptual judgment and identification. For many of the studies outlined previously and present in the literature, it is legitimate to ask whether they test *judgment* and categorization or rather what observers *see*. While it is relatively uncontroversial that judgments are cognitively penetrable, the issue is whether perception has this feature as well.

The lack of distinction between testing for perceptual judgment and testing for perception is particularly evident in the studies that purport to show emotive effects and, for this reason, the existence, extent, and significance of such effects is not well-established.[99] For other studies as well, however, the existence of a control is rare, and when it is present, the results favor a non-perceptual interpretation.[100]

In what follows, I neglect these complications and do not adjudicate the debate concerning modularity and the observation-theory distinction. I am willing to grant that, in some sense, background mental states have certain repercussions on what we see, and that these repercussions are not mere effects on judgment. Whether this amounts to admitting cognitive penetrability in perception depends on how restrictively we define it.[101] What I am interested in establishing, is whether admitting some such effects has any bearing on the plausibility of the embedded view. In order to answer this question I focus, in particular, on purported cases of penetrability by rational states, such as beliefs.

---

99. Barrick et al. 2002. Thanks to Susanna Siegel for pressing this point. See also Firestone and Scholl, forthcoming for a similar point.

100. The 'weapon bias' is a particularly good example of this. White subjects primed with the face of a black male are more likely to misidentify a briefly presented hand tool with a gun (Payne 2001, 2006). The effects could be caused by a misperception of the tool as a gun given the primed expectation. Nevertheless, two types of control suggest that the effects are due to a misclassification of what observers see (Stewart 2007, p. 15). In one experiment, confidence ratings were taken immediately after each gun/tool response. When participants responded correctly, their subjective confidence in being correct was high. When they responded incorrectly, however, their subjective confidence was low. This indicates that participants had some reason to suppose that their response was not reflective of what they saw. Along the same lines, in one study, subjects were given the opportunity to respond twice: once right after the presentation of the gun/tool, and then a second time. While they displayed a weapon bias in the first response, they corrected it in the second, making much fewer mistakes. The stereotype of a certain social category as dangerous seems to affect not what the subjects *see* but how they *classify* what they see.

101. See Macpherson 2012 and Deroy 2013 for good discussions of penetrability.

Proponents of inferentialism do not typically appeal to semantic influences in arguing for their position. They take their hypothesis to follow from considerations of performance, explanatory power, and/or computational modeling. Since I am arguing that these other reasons do not justify an inferential outlook, I now turn to cognitive penetrability as a potential source of support for it.

If we take penetrability to show that vision is reason-responsive, then we would have some motivation to suppose that vision is also not a wired and associative process. Recall that associative transitions are not breakable by logical means. Transitions between the registration of intensity changes at the retina and states that respond to edges resemble the transitions that we might instantiate when we move from tokening SALT to tokening PEPPER. These transitions are not changeable by simply presenting contrary evidence—for instance, evidence that salt and pepper do not necessarily go together.

The question is whether cases of cognitive penetrability are properly seen as cases of rational intervention of beliefs and knowledge on perception. If they are, then they would support the idea that vision is not a wired system. I now argue that we can understand these cases in a way that is compatible with EV. Embedded visual systems are biased by environmental pressure and attentional focus, and this makes them as flexible as cognitive penetrability requires.

Context-sensitivity without reason-responsiveness

Consider, first, the case of the indenting coins discussed previously (figure 4.13). This a case where completion seems to depend on known contextual information. We can imagine the visual apparatus being set to process objects as if they are complete. This, as we know from section 4.6, is plausible for independent reasons. The system is set to compute indenting coins as complete regardless of what they are penetrating. It is then exposed to information that indicates that some objects do not allow indentation. Given this evidence, the system changes the way it processes the input. It issues a representation of an incomplete object given the contrasting evidence. In so doing, the system appears to adjust to reasons.

Similarly, vision may be set to process the brightness of a face in a certain way, but by being exposed to features typical of black faces, or, more generally, to evidence that the face in question belongs to a black person, it adjusts to take this evidence into account. So the faces in figure 4.11 appear darker than they are as a function of knowledge of the category to which they belong. What we see is not a direct function of the stimulus that hits the eye, but a function of the total evidence that the visual system has. Derivatively, these studies suggest that visual processing is liable to rational intervention.

On second thought, however, this conclusion is perplexing. In order to see why this is the case, we should analyze each study that we mentioned in a bit more detail. Consider, first, the brightness illusion that we experience when we look at figure 4.11. We may think that this illusion is caused by our knowledge of the category to which the faces belong. Yet, it is strange to think of this as the cause of the illusion. It is a known and previously emphasized fact of illusions that they do not dissipate once one learns that they are illusory. In the case at hand, the illusion does not disappear by using another piece of knowledge, namely knowledge that the faces are all equally bright. Why would the visual apparatus be sensitive to one kind of evidence but not the other? Why would it be susceptible to one type of rational intervention but not the other? This is perplexing.

Equally as perplexing is the case of completion. In the indenting coin example, we have a curious effect. While the consistency of the penetrating object makes no difference to how we perceive it to be, the consistency of the penetrated object does. Again, this is perplexing. Why would one kind of rational intervention work, while the other does not?

A plausible explanation of these effects that does not appeal to rational intervention is that visual processing is sensitive to contextual features that are picked up by low-level visual states, and that it is *these* features that determine how something is seen. Vision is wired to process information depending on the features it tracks initially without instantiating an inferential transition between them. Contextual elements in figure 4.13 determine the appearance of the coin, not knowledge of the physical constitution of the brick. The tracked consistency of the brick—not beliefs about it—affects how the coin is perceived. Tracking some initial features—for instance, features typical of a soft entity—activates representations of complete (or incomplete) objects in an associative manner. Since the visual system is, and has been, exposed to soft objects that are prone to indentation, it is wired to make such objects look indented.

Similarly, in the illusion of figure 4.11 visible elements of the face—such as the shapes of the nose and mouth—rather than knowledge of the category to which they belong causes the brightness illusion. Early visual states that pick up on certain elements of the face activate associatively representations of faces with a certain brightness. This seems to better explain why the illusion does not disappear by further rational intervention. The visual system, given the features of the face, is set to process them as darker.

The further question of why vision is wired to process stereotypical black faces as dark can be answered precisely by pointing out that vision is a wired system. Having been exposed, in evolutionary history and in the observer's lifetime to faces that are darker and that also have certain features, the visual system is conditioned to process them as dark. Faces with traits typical of black faces are statistically darker than faces with features typical of white faces. Since our visual system has been exposed to this fact, we can expect it to have evolved to process faces that way, and to occasionally get things wrong.

This can change, but the change is not poised to arise through rational intervention. It is rather brought about by changing contingencies. Expose visual systems to faces that have features typical of black faces but that are not dark. Do this for a large (a very large) number of trials, and you might find, as a result, that faces with those features no longer appear dark.

We reach this same conclusion if we think of how an imaginary connectionist network would perform in this context. Networks learn to discriminate objects by developing clusters of units that are tuned to some features of the stimulus.[102] As repeatedly noted, identifying what these features are is far from easy because networks do not parse inputs into intuitive categories—for instance, mouth and nose. Repeated exposure to the stimulus, however, can cause the necessary attunement. Because of their training, networks tend to process an input that has similar superficial features in the same way. The units that pick up on those features activate automatically other units that have been activated in the past in similar circumstances. This is partly why connectionist machines are able to tolerate distortions: if the features of a novel stimulus do not deviate substantially from some standard, they process it similarly to the way they process the standard. This allows nets to often get things right. Items that have similar superficial features are, in many cases, also similar in other respects. Nevertheless, it is easy to see how this way of processing can engender error. A network that is set to process a face with features typical of black faces as dark will sometimes get things wrong. Changing its performance requires changing the environment and tuning the network differently. Rational intervention is ineffective.

The kind of attunement found in artificial networks is also found in biological neural networks, and this attunement is typically called 'imprinting.' It consists of developing structures that are sensitive to certain stimuli or parts

102. Goldstone 2003, Obermayer et al. 1995.

of stimuli for processing advantage.[103] This attunement explains why people identify items more accurately both if they have been previously exposed to them, and if the new stimulus superficially resembles previously learned ones. This same fact also engenders illusion when the superficial similarities do not stand for overall similarities.

If this is correct, then the tracked visible characteristics of the faces, not knowledge or beliefs about them, make sense of the brightness illusion illustrated by figure 4.11. By appealing to what is detected initially, and to the wired nature of vision, we also make sense of why an item shaped like a banana is seen as yellow even when it is not. We similarly make sense of why the tracked material properties of a block may have effects on amodal completion. The effects are within vision not 'top-down.' This means that some purported cases of cognitive penetrability do not show that vision is sensitive to contrary information. Somewhat ironically, they are just what we should expect if vision were wired.[104]

Does this take care of *all* of the cases introduced at the beginning of this section? It does not. In some instances, appeal to statistical regularities in the past and in the present is not sufficient. Like in the case of multi-stability, some examples of cognitive penetrability require that we appeal to the role of attention.

Semantic effects on attention

Some of the examples introduced at the beginning of this section are explainable as environmental effects on how visual processing is wired. We tend to see faces with black features as black because, in our world, faces that have those features are statistically darker than faces that have different features. Not all of the examples are explainable in this way, however. Take the case in which the brightness of an ambiguous face (middle faces in figure 4.11) is a function of the label. The same face is seen as darker if labeled 'black' and brighter if labeled 'white.'

This appears to be an instance of rational intervention. The label activates a belief that, in turn, has an effect on how we see the face. Curiously, however, one could not replace the label with another arbitrary label and obtain a change

---

103. Goldstone 2003. Training leads to changes at very early stages of perceptual processing: for instance, practice in discriminating among small visual motions alters brain potentials in primary visual cortex (Fahle and Morgan 1996; Goldstone 2003, p. 239, Schacter 1987).

104. This also means that some purported instances of penetrability are not genuine instances of cognitive penetrability on perception at all, but, as already noted, I leave this issue aside.

in perceived brightness.[105] Suppose we assign the face the label 'Asian.' It is at least dubious that this label would produce any clear effect on brightness—that is, any effect that is different from the effect that we get when the face is labeled, say, 'white.' This raises the same old puzzle: why would vision be sensitive to *some* rational interventions, but not to others? The answer seems to be, again, that it is because rational interventions are not responsible for the effects. What is?

In order to answer this question, it is useful to reflect on why assigning the label 'Asian' would not intuitively produce a significant effect. Plausibly, it would not because the face in question has no distinctive features of an Asian face. It is ambiguous between a white and a black face. Not between a white, a black, and an Asian face. Since it is the features that drive how the face is perceived, the label would not be effective. This suggests that the function of the label is primarily guiding attention—or guiding knowledge and belief that then guide attention. If a face is labeled 'black,' observers are likely to pay attention to the features of the face that are distinctive of black faces and this in turn produces a darker percept.

Observers, in other words, are trying to make the face fit the label by focusing on the features that are consistent with the label. If the face is labeled 'white' the focus is on features typical of white faces. Upon detecting the initial features, an associative visual system is conditioned to process the brightness of the face in a certain way. This produces a percept of a lighter face.[106]

In this scenario, beliefs and knowledge affect what we see only indirectly, that is, by affecting what we pay attention to. As a consequence, this is a case of rational intervention on attention, not on vision *per se*. This is a case of *biased attention*—that is, attention driven by stereotypes.

Biased attention makes sense of the studies involving anger perception as well. High-prejudiced subjects exposed to films of black faces changing in

---

105. I mean, intuitively one couldn't, because, as a matter of fact, this just hasn't been tested.

106. Researchers in this study tried to control for shifts in attention, but they controlled for the wrong thing. Their idea is that attention may be responsible for the effect because subjects tend to focus on lighter parts of white-labeled faces—such as the eyes—and on darker parts of black-labeled faces—such as the hair. This, however, is not what I am recommending. The idea is rather that the effect occurs because subjects focus on features of the face—for instance, mouth and nose—that are characteristic of white or black faces regardless of their brightness. The control by Levin and Banaji indeed confirms this hypothesis. The brightness effect shows up even if we run the study with line drawings of faces that are colored with the same shade of gray all over (Levin and Banaji 2006, experiment 3). Since the line drawings preserve the characteristic features of different faces, this experiment confirms, rather than disproves, the influence of attentional mechanisms.

expression (figure 4.12) are likely to be more alert and to focus on the features of the faces that favor a negative interpretation—that is, an interpretation of a particular face as displaying anger. Derivatively, such individuals are also more likely to judge sooner than low-prejudiced subjects that the face has changed expression.

Interestingly, biased attention still gets us biased perception. It gets us perception that is skewed to attend to certain features only, and to only notice *them*.[107] In this sense, it might also get us an interesting version of cognitive penetrability.

But biased perception does not demonstrate that vision is inferential. Subjects may see things differently as a result of differences in other mental states simply because such states determine where attention is focused. If I am skewed to focus on edges rather than on something else, then I am likely to see them because vision, picking up on discontinuities in light intensity of a certain orientation, associatively produces a representation of edges. Similarly, if I am prone to think that black people are aggressive, then I am likely to be more alert and to look for features of a face that signal anger.

Here, beliefs determine what we see, but this is hardly surprising, as these mental states have mere selective effects. They affect perception because they determine where the wired visual system focuses. As a result, they can be pernicious as they favor noticing certain elements of a visual scene over others. Nevertheless, they do not determine perception in a way that supports thinking of the visual system as an inferential system. The person who pays attention is susceptible to rational intervention, but her visual apparatus is not.

Differences in discriminative skills between novices and experts can also be ascribed to attentional differences. Knowledge and expertise help visual tuning primarily by determining the perceptual relevance of stimuli in the environment. They determine which information is important and worthy of attention and which is not.[108] Experts simply understand where it is more useful to look, and this improves their recognitional and discriminatory abilities.

This position is supported by the fact that differences between experts and novices are typically not differences in general perceptual or mnemonic skills. They are rather domain-specific advantages. This is obvious in the relatively large literature on sport performance: differences between experienced

107. Siegel 2013 also makes this point.

108. Goldstone 1998.

players and novices are largely given by being able to anticipate relevant events. This is done, for example, by observing initial segments of an opponent's gesture in throwing a ball.[109]

Similarly, in chick sexing, novices do not know where to look. This is confirmed by the fact that simple training, consisting of an instruction that specifies the location and kind of diagnostic features, increases novices' performance, making it similar to that of experts even in the errors that both groups commit.

Analyzing the eye movements of chess masters yields similar results. Masters look at how pieces attack and defend each other, a capacity that is likely involved in their ability to see pieces in chunks.[110] Finally, experienced radiologists process X-ray images better than do new students primarily by devoting processing resources to features that are distinctive. Their attention is quickly captured by unexpected elements. For expert radiologists, a single eye fixation is sufficient to detect and identify major pathological features with 70% accuracy.[111]

If this is right, then in many cases, we can explain semantic effects on perception as semantic effects on attention. This, combined with appeal to environmental conditions, accounts for purported cases of cognitive penetrability in a fully embedded framework.

4.9 Conclusion

This chapter showed that a number of visual cases that are thought to be problematic for direct accounts of vision are readily explainable if we are careful about the claims that embedded theorists are committed to.

What should be clear from this discussion is that the embedded view is an explanatorily powerful empirical hypothesis. I concluded the chapter by showing that the embedded framework is compatible with, and explains, instances of cognitive penetration, where vision appears to be sensitive to other psychological states. If this is true, then EV is plausible on both theoretical and empirical grounds. I conclude the case in its favor by showing, in the next chapter, that EV is also compatible with computationalism.

---

109. Abernethy 1991, Abernethy et al. 1994.

110. Simon and Barenfeld 1969.

111. Kundel and Nodine 1975, Myles-Worsley et al. 1988.

5

Computation

My point will be that not only considered action, but also learning and perception, must surely be viewed as based upon computational processes; and, once again, no computation without representation.

(FODOR 1975, p. 34.)

Even such programs as the Gibsonian theory of perception are ultimately compatible with minimal computationalism. If perception turns out to work as the Gibsonians imagine, it will still be mediated by causal mechanisms, and the mechanisms will be expressible in an appropriate computational form. That expression may look very unlike a traditional computational theory of perception, but it will be computational nevertheless.

(CHALMERS 2011, p. 355)

5.1 Introduction

Chapter 4 showed that the embedded view has the resources to explain a number of visual phenomena that are presumably troublesome for direct accounts. If the considerations from chapter 3 are cogent, then EV has been shown to be more plausible than cognitive competitors on both theoretical and evidential grounds. This chapter concludes the case in favor of the embedded view by discussing whether (and the sense in which) it is compatible with computationalism.

Not everybody accepts the computational theory of mind (CTM), the idea that mental processes are computational. As a consequence, this chapter may be of interest only to those who do. Nevertheless, three issues should raise independent curiosity for what is covered here.

The first issue concerns the fact that computational models of visual activity are widely used in cognitive science and they are partly responsible for some of the success of the science.[1] It is thus independently interesting to see how the embedded view fares vis à vis computationalism, and what consequences accepting it has for CTM.

The second issue is that ecological and embedded accounts of perception are often taken to be at odds with computationalism. Gibson himself, writing before more recent developments in computer science, rejected a computational framework. As I argue in this chapter, however, there is no incompatibility between computationalism and embedded approaches. Indeed, it is precisely by reflecting on more recent computational systems, and on how to understand the notion of computation that we can develop views like the embedded view.

The final issue concerns the relation between inferentialism and *classical* computational models. One may take vision to be inferential not only because it encodes some implicit assumptions (as we have reason to suppose that inferentialists about vision do) but also because it manipulates representations that have propositional format. This way of understanding the visual process would be supported by the classical way of understanding computations. If vision were computational in the classical sense, then it would be a transition between representations that look like symbols. The symbols would have syntactic structure and combinatorial syntax and semantics, resembling words and sentences of a language.

In this picture, the visual process would be a process that approximates an inference in a number of relevant respects. The process would instantiate *logical*, inference-like transitions between states that look like premises and states that look like conclusions. For this reason, classical computationalism was once a primary reason to accept inferential accounts of perception.[2] It is then interesting to go back to some of the motivations for accepting classicism and discuss whether they apply to the visual case. Since the embedded view favors non-classical ways of understanding computations we should discuss how EV fares in relation to pro-classicism arguments.

To summarize what this chapter accomplishes, I argue that the embedded view is compatible with the computational theory of mind broadly understood, and that we have little reason to suppose that classicism is the only good model of visual processing. To establish the first point, I argue that there are perfectly

1. Perhaps computational models are also responsible for some of the failures of cognitive science, but this would be the conclusion of an argument that I do not have space to reproduce and discuss here.

2. Ullman 1979.

legitimate models of computation that do not describe them as regimented operations on symbols or representations. Connectionist networks are prime examples of such computations, but even more traditional digital computations do not require representations.[3] Section 5.2 is devoted to explaining this point.

I then move on to argue that denying that the visual system performs computations, in the classical sense is justified by the lack of reasons to see visual and sensory states as propositionally structured, and it does not amount to rejecting classical CTM altogether. We need only maintain that the computational theory of mind, traditionally understood, is true of other mental processes. Section 5.3 is devoted to explaining why this is a legitimate and beneficial position to take.

A final word about the chapter. In closing this book, I do not propose a novel theory of computation, and I do not survey, in any detail, the rich literature on computationalism that developed in the last thirty or so years. My intent is more modest. I aim to show that, if you like computationalism, then you can accept EV because the present state of research on the notion of computation indicates that embedded visual systems are computational. In doing this, the chapter relies on the work of others in the field whose research developed independently of the need to defend a specific non-inferential perspective on vision.[4] With this, I hope to make the embedded view appealing to a diverse audience.

5.2 Computation without representation

Proponents of cognitive accounts of perception often see their commitment to the idea that vision is cognitive as one and the same with their adherence to the computational theory of mind.[5] This is because, at a minimum, computations are thought to be operations over representational states, so any computational process is *ipso facto* a process that involves representations.

Direct and embedded models of vision do not accord with computational outlooks so described. Since the embedded view does not conceive of visual

3. Piccinini 2008a.

4. I use, in particular, the work of Gualtiero Piccinini and David Chalmers. See also Wilson (Wilson 2004, ch. 7), and Haugeland (Haugeland 1998, ch. 9) for attempts to formulate non-classical accounts of computation.

5. Fodor 1984, Fodor and Pylyshyn 1981, Gregory 1970, Marr 1982, Palmer 1999, p. 71, Rock 1983.

processes as operations on representations, it seems to be openly incompatible with CTM. If we were to accept the further premise that computationalism is the only plausible and scientifically respectable account of mental activity,[6] we would have an explicit argument against the embedded view.

A natural way to respond to this argument is to simply deny that computationalism is true with respect to vision. If the embedded account is at odds with computationalism, and EV is right, then so much the worse for computationalism; vision is not a computational process after all.

Although quite blunt, this response is right in one respect. If we take computationalism in a restricted sense, then visual processes are not computational processes. Section 5.3 explains why this is not so bad after all. In the present section, however, I want to show that embedded accounts are compatible with computationalism. This is because we can formulate a notion of computation that does not individuate computations by appeal to representations, and that seems better responsive to how the notion is used in computer science. There are computations that do not consist in the regimented manipulation of representations. As a matter of fact, computations may be carried out by systems that do not represent at all. Embedded visual systems are examples of such systems.

Classical computations: rules and language

Like in the case of the notion of representation, accounts of computation vary in how *committal* they are. Classical views are committal. According to such views, computations are operations over linguistic symbols, and transitions between the symbols are regulated by encoded algorithms.[7] There are, as a result, two important components of computations according to classicism: linguistic symbols and sets of rules.

In concrete computing systems, the symbols of classical computations are given by strings of 0s and 1s and they are instantiated, or realized, by some macroscopic state of a computing device—for instance, a type of electrical state of part of a computer.[8] What is particularly important about the symbols in classical computations is that they are *linguistic*. Like words of a language, the symbols have syntax and semantics and they can combine and recombine to form 'strings.' Strings have a sentence-like form, being evaluable for truth and

6. Fodor 1975.

7. Fodor 1975, Pylyshyn 1984.

8. Piccinini and Scarantino 2011, p. 26.

displaying genuine predication. The strings are not mere 'lists of features' but symbolic structures with sentential format.[9] Importantly, strings in classical computations have a combinatorial structure. What the strings mean systematically depends on what the component symbols mean. Linguistic symbols are thus the basic vehicles of classical computations.

Algorithms regulate the operations on the symbols and the strings of symbols (the sentences). An algorithm is, in the classicist paradigm, an "effective, step-by-step procedure" to manipulate strings of symbols and to "produce a result within finitely many steps."[10] Classical algorithms are sets of rules that guide a computation and that produce a desired output in a finite and discrete number of stages. In classical computers, the algorithms are typically encoded in a certain component of the computational system, the concrete program. Encoded rules may be implemented in binary strings that are physically realized in some part of the computational device.[11] In this picture, computers are rule-following machines.

Because of their commitment to both symbolic (representational) states and encoded principles of processing, classical computations pair up well with inferential accounts of vision.[12] Jerry Fodor and Zenon Pylyshyn, for example, write:

> The current Establishment theory (sometimes referred to as the "information processing" view) is that perception depends, in several respects presently to be discussed, upon inferences. Since inference is a process in which premises are displayed and consequences derived, and since that takes time, it is part and parcel of the information processing view that there is an intrinsic connection between perception and memory. And since, finally, the Establishment holds that the psychological mechanism of inference is the transformation of mental representations, it follows that perception is in relevant respects a computational process.
>
> (Fodor and Pylyshyn 1981, p. 140)

9. Fodor and Pylyshyn 1988.

10. Piccinini and Scarantino 2011, p. 9.

11. Piccinini 2008a, p. 214.

12. Marr 1982, p. 36.

The classical way of understanding computations has several advantages. A general one is that classical models offer a way to explain, in a mechanistic spirit, how mental states can have content and also be causally efficacious in the production of behavior in a way that seems to depend on the content itself. This was thought to be an insight of Copernican magnitude since, prior to the advent of computers, explaining how a mechanical system could be sensitive to semantic elements was utterly puzzling.[13] This advantage is not exclusive to classical models, however. All computational systems, when they manipulate representational or contentful states, also have this advantage.

A more specific bonus point of classicism is that it is perceived to be the only way to explain the productivity and systematicity of thought (more on this in section 5.3). This virtue of classicism comes from identifying mental representations with linguistic symbols that can combine and recombine in lawful ways to form sentence-like structures (thoughts).

Reflection on other types of computers and on the practice of computer science, however, reveals that classical computations are only one kind of computational systems.

Computation without rules

It was first noted that encoding algorithms is not required to define a computation.[14] There are computers that operate on symbolic elements, but that do not execute algorithms. They are rather 'hardwired' or 'wired' to do what they do.

In previous chapters, I often used the example of connectionist networks as systems that do not follow rules, but, as we noted back in section 2.2, even more traditional computers can be wired systems. Arithmetic logic units are common examples. They operate in a discrete fashion on states that stand for mathematical elements, but they conform to principles that they do not encode. We can *describe* the units as following the rules of, say, addition, but the units do not instantiate any structure that encodes the rules. Arithmetic logic units are simply made to transition between symbolic elements (numbers) in a way that conforms to addition without executing a procedure for adding.

---

13. Fodor 1975.

14. See Cummins 1983, pp. 44–51 for an early discussion of this point. Thanks to an anonymous referee for the pointer.

It is now generally accepted in computer science that, in principle, anything that can be computed with encoded rules can also be computed by wired systems. In practice, task demands—such as fast flexibility and durability—can make one type of computation preferable to the other. Nevertheless, as far as the notion of computation goes, we have no trouble recognizing that wired systems are computational.[15]

Computation without linguistic symbols

Computations do not need encoded algorithms; neither do they require linguistic units. Computations can occur between map-like structures and/or between lists of symbols that do not combine to form sentence-like aggregates. The 'strings' of computations may lack both linguistic form (failing to resemble genuine sentences) and a combinatorial syntax and semantics.

Computational models of navigation in probabilistic robotics, for example, employ 'cognitive maps' that have geometric rather than linguistic structure. The units of computation in these models look like lists of spatial properties and relations and they do not resemble sentences. Such robotic models demonstrate the possibility of computations without genuine linguistic constituents.[16]

The impression that computations have to occur between linguistic elements is invited by a certain way of understanding digital computation. Digital computation is a more general notion than classical computation as described earlier. Digital computation typically consists of operations on strings of elements, called 'digits' according to rules defined over the digits (but not necessarily encoded within the digital machine).[17] A digit is roughly a state that, in a system, can be reliably distinguished from other states and treated as the same in different contexts. It may be implemented by a voltage level or, in computational models of brain activity, by a neuronal spike.[18] Digits

---

15. Thanks to an anonymous referee for making this point clear. Piccinini also notices that, even in cases in which a computer encodes an algorithm, the algorithm may not have any 'proper semantics.' It may have a type of 'internal semantics,' that is, it may refer to the internal language and operations of the computer (Piccinini 2008a, pp. 214–215). The algorithmic rules may stand for commands that do not reflect external facts or regularities. This is an interesting point, but I leave it undiscussed. What is relevant to my thesis is that computers don't need to encode algorithms at all in order to be computers. They can simply conform to algorithms without following them.

16. Rescorla 2009a.

17. Piccinini and Scarantino 2011, p. 7.

18. Piccinini and Bahar 2012.

may appear to implement linguistic representations, because, like letters or words, they can be seen as elements that can be concatenated into strings and distinguished from each other inside the string.

At the abstract level, digits are typically labeled with numbers—the 0s and 1s typical of computation. The numbers or strings of numbers can, in turn, be labeled with words of a language. This allows programmers to write—in abstract—how the digits should enter in, and be manipulated by, the computer so that the computer can perform a certain function. It is easy to assign both a specific meaning and a linguistic label to each of the digits and then see them as linguistic elements.

Contrary to what classical models hold, however, there is nothing mandatory about this way of treating digits. Digits do not need to be labeled with linguistic symbols. They can be seen to instantiate maps or images or spatial locations or whatever else explains and describes what the computational system does. There are digital computations performed over words of a language, and there are equally as respectable digital computations that operate on mere lists of spatial properties and relations, or on maps, or on images, or on nonsense elements. It is simply not necessary to view the digits as elements of a language and/or to program a computer so that it manipulates linguistic elements.

We then moved from a very *committal* way of understanding computations to a more *deflated* notion. According to classicism, computers are distinctive in both employing linguistic representations and encoding rules of processing. We first saw that encoded rules are not needed to individuate computations, and we later appreciated that linguistic symbols are also not needed. Computational transitions need not be inferential. They may be associative transitions where a cognitive map encoded by a digit activates another in virtue of closeness.

I now introduce an even more deflated way of understanding computations. According to such understanding, the notion of representation, linguistic or not, is not needed at all to define a computation. To see computational systems as also trading in representations is sometimes useful and can certainly be done, but it is an additional and non mandatory claim.

Computation without representation

In order to see that representations are not needed to individuate computational processes, we should start by recognizing that the digits in a computer do not need to stand for something in order to count as digits. As long as a state is distinguishable from others in different contexts, and as long as it enters into lawful transitions with other states, it is a digit even if it has no semantic interpretation.

Just as there are digital computations that occur between map-like structures, there are also digital computations that operate over strings that are not meaningful at all—for example, strings labeled as 'r%h@.'[19] Digital computations do not need to be defined over meaningful elements that inform or that represent. The strings of digits can be given a semantic interpretation by the programmer—that is, they can be interpreted as standing for numerals, or for chess moves, or for light-intensity values—but they need not do so in order to figure in perfectly legitimate computations.[20] As long as a system is properly described as operating in a regimented fashion over digits, then the system is computing digitally even if it does not represent at all.

Notice further that if we accept the distinction between representational and tracking states, then a system that processes information is not thereby a system that processes representations. The digits in a computer may be states that co-vary with environmental elements—thereby carrying information about them—and they may enter into encapsulated transitions without being representations. A computational system built to act like a retina will have digits that act like retinal states. Such states carry information and track, but they are not representations.

This point allows us to recognize that, in some cases, computations may be usefully individuated in terms of informational content[21] while also not requiring appeal to representations. Most computationalists are in favor of drawing some sort of distinction between representational states and states that merely correlate with environmental elements.[22] It seems to follow from this that an information-processing system is not, *ipso facto*, a representation-processing system.

That representations and computations do not go together is further illustrated by less traditional types of computing systems, such as connectionist networks. In a network, it is hard to identify digits, and consequently it is hard to assign a semantic interpretation to the internal states of the connectionist machine. Networks can be seen as digital in a very minimal sense because

19. Piccinini and Scarantino 2011, p. 12.

20. Piccinini 2008a, p. 211.

21. Rescorla 2012.

22. Piccinini and Scarantino 2011.

only their inputs and their outputs are digits. They are input/output digital systems (I/O systems).[23]

Connectionist nets do not perform operations of 'symbol manipulation' in any sense. They instantiate evolutions of weights and activations. As we saw in previous chapters, networks that use back-propagation learn their tasks by adjusting the strength of the connections between the units. This is done until the networks output the right response when exposed to a large set of training material. In artificial nets, a program can be written that adjusts the weights in this way, and it is yet unclear what allows weight adjustment in non-artificial neural nets. After the training period, however, networks are typically able to detect what they are designed to detect without manipulating symbols, linguistic or of other kinds.

In networks of this kind, the input and the output units may be identifiable as digits, but the outputs are not produced by following step-by-step procedures, or rules, and by going through internal discrete stages. Those who program connectionist networks often try to give input and output units a semantic interpretation. This may be particularly easy in the case of the output. We may, for example, set a network to output a certain value—for example, the vector $< 1, 1, 1, 1 >$—whenever a mine echo is present. As a consequence, a certain activation of the output units may be seen as standing for the presence of mine echoes. Notice, however, that this encoding of mine echoes would be highly 'distributed' and non-symbolic. We would not know, for example, which part of the output stands for 'mine' and which part stands for 'echo.' In general, this question makes little sense in the case of networks, because their output is a level of activation that does not come packaged in symbols.

We may also try to assign a semantic interpretation to the input and hidden units, seeing them as tuned to specific environmental parameters. This identification, however, is often hard and arbitrary. The problem is that it is not clear what environmental features, if any, the input and the hidden units track. Network units do not respond individually to specific inputs. They may be tuned to specific elements, like in imprinting (chapter 4), but these elements are not intuitive and easily identifiable—that is, they are not as simple as, say, 'edges.' This is why networks are typically seen as operating over 'subsymbolic states.'

Moreover, although we could ascribe content to the subsymbolic states, such ascription is not necessary to think of the network as a computing

23. Piccinini 2011, p. 234.

system, or to understand how the network carries out its task. What the programmer typically does is adjust the level of activation of the units to get the desired response. The concern is *not* with what the units stand for but rather with how active they should be in order to produce the response that we want—that is, the output vector that we want. Accordingly, networks that reduce error are able to produce the appropriate digital output through a series of internal transformations that need not have a semantic interpretation.[24]

The idea is not that a semantic interpretation of networks and of other computing systems is in principle inappropriate; rather, the idea is that it is in practice not needed to individuate the computation. In the case of the connectionist nets I described, this idea is even more vivid than in the case of more standard digital computers because the distributed nature of the states of the network make the semantic interpretation difficult. This motivates some recent skeptical arguments against the utility of mental representations. The skeptical thought is as follows: if every mental process is better modeled by connectionism, then this makes trouble for the thesis that mentality consists in operations on representations.[25] But even if we leave aside connectionism and consider more traditional digital computers, we should realize that understanding the digits as representational elements is not mandatory.

We thus need to detach the notion of a computational system from the notion of a system that represents. A system may be computational without representing anything. Views of computation that recognize this point can be labeled *deflationary views* and, like deflationary views of representation, they come in different degrees. We should conclude this section by briefly surveying two types of deflationary accounts together with their virtues and vices.

24. The fact that connectionist networks do not follow algorithms and do not operate over digits may raise some questions concerning whether we should call such computing systems 'digital.' This may be mostly a verbal dispute. If the inputs and outputs are digits, then the label 'I/O digital' seems appropriate. On the other hand, there are computational systems that are not digital even in this minimal sense. These are analogue computers (Piccinini and Scarantino 2011, p. 11). The notion of computation is wider than the notion of digital computation, which in turn is wider than the notion of classical computation.

25. Ramsey 1997, 2007. Here, I do not need to assess this debate. The question of whether *all* mental processes are better modeled by connectionism is an empirical issue that goes beyond the scope of this book. We can simply recognize that networks help us see that the notion of computation and the notion of representation do not go together.

Minimalism

Deflationism with respect to computation, as described in this section, holds that defining what a computation is does not require appeal to representation. There are different types of deflationism. At the minimal end of the spectrum, a system performs computations simply when the system's causal organization maps a computational description.[26] In this minimal view, the causal structure of the system mirrors the formal structure of the computation, where this mirroring means that there is a sort of isomorphism between the two. The steps specified in the computational description correspond accurately to the succession of steps that occur in the physical system. Following its main proponents, we may call this view *minimalism*.

Minimalism is often deemed unappealing because it appears to trivialize the notion of computation and to invite pancomputationalism, the view that all systems in the environment compute (unsurprisingly a problem similar to the one that plagues deflationary accounts of representation). Since, according to minimalism, a system is computational just in case there is a mapping from a formal description to its causal organization, it seems that everything, including rocks, would be a very simple computational system.[27] All we need to recognize that a system such as a rock is computational is to map an initial physical state onto an initial formal state of a computation, and then map successive states of the system onto successive states of the computation.

This is obviously a problem and an important issue for minimalism because the idea that minds are distinctive in performing computational operations is supposed to be a substantive hypothesis. Appeal to computation is supposed to illuminate what minds do that is *different* from what other things do. If every system performs computations, however, then appeal to this idea would seem to lose explanatory power. The mind would be computational just like everything else.

One of the advantages of resorting to representations to define computations is precisely that this appeal restricts the number of systems that are able to genuinely compute, since it restricts it to the number of systems that are also able to represent. It effectively distinguishes computing systems (like, presumably, minds) from systems that may be complex but that do not compute (rocks, planets, and stomachs). Although the latter may have

---

26. Chalmers 2011.

27. Putnam 1988.

states that interact in various lawful ways, such states are not symbolic or representational.[28]

As we saw, the practice of computer science does not warrant the view that computations are distinctive in employing representations. We need a different way to restrict the notion of computation.

Minimalism holds that every system implements (at the very least) one computation because every physical system implements a finite state *automaton* with a single internal state.[29] Additionally, most systems might implement a simple two-state computation as they instantiate lawful transitions between two states. Nevertheless, minimalists can retain some substance for their position by pointing out that not every system implements any given computation. Complex computations require fairly complex causal organizations such that very few physical systems implement them.

Minimalists remark, in particular, that the mapping of formal states onto physical states requires there to be a reliable, counterfactual-supporting connection between two (or more) states of the system. What this means is that for there to be a mapping it is not sufficient that, say, state *A* is followed by state *B* at one time. What's required is rather that the transition from *A* to *B* is reliable and counterfactual-supporting where, if the system were to be in state *A*, it would transit to state *B*. Complex computations that involve many such transitions are instantiated by only a small number of physical systems.

This explains why rocks and planets, although instantiating *some* computations, are not computational systems in any more interesting sense. The notion of computation, in and of itself, may not be illuminating in understanding what is distinctive of minds, but the notion of *complex* computation is.

Additionally, minimalism holds that not every system has the capacities that it has *in virtue* of instantiating a computation. Stomachs, for instance, may be fairly complex computational systems, instantiating lawful transitions between states that are describable by a program. Instantiating a complex computation is not sufficient for them to do what they do, however. That the stomach instantiates a computation is irrelevant to it performing digestion; certain chemical reactions are supposedly also required.

By contrast, the substantive hypothesis, in the case of minds, is that it is in virtue of instantiating a complex computation that minds have the capacities

---

28. Fodor 1975, n. 15.

29. Chalmers 2911, p. 331.

that they do. This is called, by Chalmers, the thesis of 'computational sufficiency.'[30]

Whether we accept this thesis or not, the preceding discussion shows that minimalists can appeal to sufficiency and complexity to retain their minimal view while preserving a substantive explanatory role for computation in theories of mind. If minimalism is right, then accepting the embedded view is compatible with accepting a computational approach to the study of vision. Embedded visual systems instantiate transitions that can be mapped by a formal or computational description. Many, however, find minimalism and the pancomputationalism that comes with it unappealing.

Non-minimal deflationism

A less deflationary proposal than minimalism is that a computational system is a particular kind of functionally organized system. As the name suggests, functionally organized systems are systems organized into components that have a certain function.[31] Both traditional and I/O digital computers have parts that are distinguished *not* by their physical properties, but by the job that they perform within the computer. They may have input components, processing units, storage units and output components.

Additionally, according to this deflationary but non-minimal position, computers are a special kind of functional mechanisms. They are distinctive because they manipulate states in virtue of certain properties of the states—for example, in virtue of the voltage level instantiated by the state—and in a way that can be accurately described by rules. That the states stand for something else, represent, or even just carry information is not needed to individuate the computation. Neither is it needed that the rules that describe the computation are followed or executed by the functional system.

Deflationary positions of this kind differ from minimalist positions because they add further conditions—for instance, functional organization—to restrict computations without appealing to semantic ideas. Appeal to functional decomposition is thought to prevent rocks and planets from performing any computations (even very simple ones) as these systems do not break down into parts that are individuated by the function they perform. The notion of function (especially in its teleological form) has no place in

30. See Chalmers 2011.

31. Piccinini 2007, 2011.

explaining what many systems do, thus restricting the set of systems that are properly seen as computing.

Further, stomachs are ruled out as computational systems in the digital sense by the appeal to the capacity to (1) identify digits—that is, states that can be distinguished from others in different contexts; and (2) the ability to see those states as persisting through a process. In the process of digestion, we seem unable to identify states that can be distinguished from others in different contexts, and that can be combined into strings. It is also difficult to see how different states of the digestive process persist through the process itself.

The existence of analogue, non-digital computers may be a problem for this way of understanding computations in relation to stomachs, but I do not want to linger on this problem. What is important, for present purposes, is that there are viable ways to restrict the notion of computation in both minimalist and other deflationary accounts without appeal to the notion of representation. If a system is decomposed into functional parts, and processes or produces digits according to rules that the machine is wired to conform to, then it performs computations even if it does not trade in representations. Again, the claim is not that it is never useful, illuminating, or appropriate to see the digits as representational elements (or to build machines that encode their principles of operation). The claim is rather (and simply) that it is not mandatory to do so.

This result introduces interesting questions concerning the interplay between computation, representation, and theories of mind. Those who believe that computation is sufficient to explain cognition may also think that the notion of representation is not central to explain how the mind works.[32] Those who, by contrast, suppose that intentionality is the central aspect of the mind are either skeptical of computational accounts,[33] or point out that computation in cognitive psychology and artificial intelligence (AI) is often individuated by appeal to semantics—that is, either by appeal to informational states or by appeal to representations.[34]

What is relevant is that accepting the embedded view does not commit us to rejecting computationalism about vision. If computational systems are functionally organized mechanisms whose operations are accurately mapped

32. Stich 1983.

33. Most notably Searle 1980.

34. Rescorla 2014.

by programs, and whose internal states are manipulated given some distinctive properties of the states, then embedded visual systems are computational. They are functionally organized systems (having input components, output components, and processing components) and they appear to manipulate states in a way that can be described by rules. As a matter of fact, low-level states may respond selectively to the environment and carry information about it, but the fact that they do is quite irrelevant to judging whether visual systems perform computations. They perform computations because of the other structural features that they have.

The further question of whether visual systems are better modeled by standard digital computers or by connectionist networks is an open empirical question. For argumentative purposes, I have been relying heavily on work on artificial nets to support the embedded view. Perhaps a bit surprisingly, however, a more traditional digital computer that does not follow an algorithm and that does not operate on linguistic structures can also be a good model of embedded seeing.

Given this conclusion, let us take stock and go back to our initial problem. A potential argument against the embedded view holds that computationalism is the only viable way to understand mental states and processes. Since vision is a mental process we should understand it as computational. Computations (*as per* classicism) consist in operations on linguistic representations in virtue of encoded rules. The embedded view does not conceive of visual processes as operations on linguistic representations in virtue of encoded rules. Thus, we should reject the embedded view.

We can now see that this argument relies on an overly narrow, and ultimately mistaken, account of computation. It may be true that computationalism is the only game in town; but, properly understood, it is perfectly compatible with EV.

Those unsatisfied with a situated account of vision may, however, reason as follows. While compatible with computationalism more generally construed, the embedded view is incompatible with at least one kind of computation, classical computation. It is this type of computation that is the only game in town. If we do not think of mental processes as operations regulated by encoded assumptions, and over vehicles that can combine to form language-like structures, then we do not have a good account of mental processes.[35]

---

35. Fodor 1975, Fodor and Pylyshyn 1988.

The next section is devoted to showing that this type of reasoning is also flawed. We have little reason to suppose that classical computation is the only viable option when it comes to explaining perception.

5.3 Seeing is not believing

The previous section showed that the embedded view is compatible with computationalism properly construed and that classicism, the view that is sometimes associated with inferential accounts of vision, describes only one—and relatively narrow—type of computation. Nevertheless, we may object that it is precisely *classicism* that we should not give up. You may accept that vision is inferential because it is a process that happens over states that have linguistic format, and you may accept this because you may think that this is the only way to make sense of mental processes more generally. Vision resembles an inference because it involves a transition between some sentence-like states to others in a premise-conclusion fashion.

What motivations do we have to accept the view that perception requires explanation in terms of classical computations? Those who believe that mental activity has to be understood on the model of classicism often make reference to the notions of productivity and systematicity. In explaining these two features of thought we seem bound to admit that psychological transitions occur between internal states that have linguistic format.[36]

This section aims to show that this argument against the embedded view and in favor of classicism does not work. We may have reasons to prefer classicism in explaining higher-order mental processes, but such reasons do not straightforwardly apply to the perceptual case. This is because the kind of productivity and systematicity that we see in perception can be explained without thinking of sensory and perceptual states as linguistically structured. I start the section by noticing a respect in which EV and classicism are compatible. I then move on to show that *perceptual* productivity and systematicity can be explained in an embedded framework.

Scruffy mental life

In a recent article, Andy Clark reminds us of a distinction between two personality types in theorizing about the mind.[37] *Neats* believe "in a few very general,

36. Fodor and Pylyshyn 1988.

37. Clark 2012, p. 193.

truth-conducive principles underlying intelligence," while *scruffies* see intelligence as "arising from a varied bag of tricks." We can put this distinction to a slightly different use in the present context to differentiate those who suppose that a single overarching computational framework will explain different mental processes (the neats) from those who deny that this is likely to happen (the scruffies).

I am inclined to side with the scruffies. Accepting the embedded view does not commit one to rejecting classicism in all of its instances, and this is a *good* thing. There may be mental processes that are best understood as classical computations, and we can admit this while holding that vision is embedded rather than cognitive. We need only maintain that the classical computational theory of mind is true of other mental activities.

This approach seems to rid us of a pernicious assumption that is reminiscent of a certain Cartesian way of looking at the mind. In the second Meditation, Descartes remarks that perceiving (*sentire*) is nothing other than thinking.[38] Although Descartes' reasons for this conclusion were different from those of contemporary computationalists, we can point out that thinking requires representational structures that are not needed in perceiving. Since the two mental processes are different, the idea that the same computational theory should explain both is not warranted.

Proponents of the classical computational theory of mind have argued that classical computationalism is the only viable option for explaining choosing, concept learning, and perceiving.[39] Ironically, it was thought that the classical framework was better at explaining perception than higher-order cognition.[40] Nonetheless, since perceiving, choosing, and learning are very different competences, we should not be so confident that a single theory can be used to cover all of them. Different mental processes may require different procedures.

That this is a legitimate position to hold is somewhat confirmed by the fact that the reasons that are typically offered for deeming classicism the only plausible account of mental activity do not easily apply to perception. These reasons have to do primarily with two seemingly distinctive features of thought: systematicity and productivity. I discuss them, and how they show up in perception, in the following subsection.

---

38. Descartes 1641.

39. Fodor 1975.

40. Fodor 1983.

Productivity and systematicity in perception

Productivity and systematicity are both presented as properties of thinking. Productivity consists of the fact that thinking agents, despite being finite, appear capable of producing novel thoughts in infinite number. Systematicity is, in turn, the fact that the ability to have certain thoughts is related to the ability to have certain others.[41]

These features seem to require that mental processes occur over states that have linguistic form. A potentially infinite number of new thoughts may be produced by combining simple thoughts (atomic symbols) that one already has. From a finite 'vocabulary' we derive an infinite ability.

Individuals faced with novel circumstances, for instance, are typically able to think about them, and make decisions in them, because they can combine old thoughts to form new ones that apply in the novel situation. Further, individuals can consider options in thought that they have never previously entertained.

If we think in linguistic symbols that are easily put together into meaningful structures, then this capacity is readily explained. If, on the other hand, we think that mental representations lack linguistic structure (an accusation that connectionist representations—being distributed and non-syntactic—often face) then it is a mystery how finite beings could produce potentially infinite new thoughts. Every new thought in a connectionist net is a new network configuration and presumably there are only finitely many configurations. Additionally, every new thought, lacking genuine syntactic constituents, is not produced by combining old thoughts and it potentially bears little resemblance to them.

Classicism appears to also have little trouble explaining systematicity. The ability to have certain thoughts is related to the ability to have certain others because similar thoughts have common constituents. The thought 'Chase loves Julio' has similar semantic and syntactic parts to the thought 'Julio loves Chase' and 'Chase loves Chase,' so classicism predicts that an individual who is capable of entertaining one of these thoughts will also be able to entertain the others. If, however, we think that thoughts do not have linguistic parts, then we are not able to predict this systematicity. On the contrary, we should

---

41. Fodor and Pylyshyn 1988 is the *locus classicus* for arguments that favor classicism by using productivity and systematicity. Strictly speaking, systematicity is the fact that the ability to have certain thoughts is *intrinsically* related to the ability to have certain others, but since I am not clear on what 'intrinsically' means in this context, I work with a more generic definition.

find punctuate minds—minds that can only think one of these thoughts—as completely unsurprising.

Defenders of non-classical models of computation, and of corresponding accounts of mental activity, react to these considerations in different ways. Some point out that it is dubious that thinking has the features outlined previously. Others argue that non-classical architectures are capable of accounting for such features.[42] In what follows, I pursue briefly this latter line of reasoning. I show that the type of productivity and systematicity that we encounter in perception is explainable without appeal to sensory and perceptual states that have sentence-like structure. This may suggest a more general strategy to reject linguistic representations in accounts of psychological competences. I do not pursue this more general strategy, however, as I am interested solely in the perceptual case.

To be clear, the argument is that, while it may be intuitive or even—to some—obvious that the productivity and systematicity of thought requires thinking in linguistic format, this is not as intuitive or obvious in the case of perception. The kind of systematicity and productivity that we find in perceptual states is seemingly explainable by appeal to map-like or list-like representations, and it is not obvious that such representations are linguistic. Thus, defenders of classicism would need additional arguments to conclude that perceptual and sensory states are sententially structured—for example, arguments to suppose that map-like representations are linguistic at base.

Consider productivity first. Fodor himself admits that the productivity argument is debatable,[43] and notice that, as a capacity for producing potentially infinite new mental states, it is not clear how it applies to perception. Perceptions are not produced by combining old perceptual or sensory states in the absence of input—like new thoughts may be produced by combining old ones. Rather, perceptions are produced by being responsive to the world and having new encounters with it. It is true that if one is able to perceive red in one context, then she is also typically able to perceive it in a new context. This capacity, however, is diagnostic of an ability to respond to similar environmental inputs in similar ways. It is not due to the ability to combine basic mental representations in novel guises. Productivity seems to require a generative ability that is distinctive of thought—and perhaps of other higher-order mental abilities—not of sensation and of perception.

42. Chalmers 1992, 1993, Smolensky 1988a, Van Gelder 1990.

43. Fodor 1987a, p. 148.

Perception is productive in the sense that it can discriminate 'productive properties'—that is, properties such that, if one is capable of detecting them, then one is also capable of detecting novel stimuli that instantiate them.[44] As proponents of inferential accounts of vision grant, however, productive properties can be discriminated by systems that do not perform classical computations, and in fact by systems that are mere resonators to physical parameters.[45] All it takes to be able to detect productive properties of certain kinds is to have, or acquire, the ability to respond consistently to similar inputs. Accordingly, our capacity to see certain colors in many displays is no evidence for the need to treat vision as a classical computation.

Something similar can be said of systematicity. It is at first hard to understand what systematicity means in relation to perception. In the case of thought, systematicity manifests as the fact that the ability to have certain thoughts is related to the ability to have certain others. It is hard to see what the perceptual analogue of this is, however. Is it that the ability to see a red cube is related to the ability to see a cube red? It is dubious that there is any difference between these two states at the level of perceptual content.

The hurdle seems to be that, in order for us to understand systematicity in relation to perception, we would have to already accept that perceptual states have a thought-like form—a form that involves, say, predication and a subject-object structure. In this case, we could, speaking loosely, move the subject and the predicate around and account for why different perceptions, having common elements, are related. But this is not an assumption that we can freely make in the present dialectical situation.

Perhaps, an example of systematicity in perception is given by perceptual states that represent relational properties. If one is able to see the square above the rectangle, she is also typically able to see the rectangle above the square. As in the case of productivity, however, this perceptual ability is seemingly explained by the ability to discriminate spatial relations. This ability can be achieved by employing map-like representations, without needing linguistic ones. 'Square above triangle' can be encoded in a map rather than in a sentence.

While maps may have, in some sense, syntactic parts—for instance, markers that are spatially arranged in a certain way and that can be labeled with symbols—they do not resemble linguistic descriptions in other respects. Maps

44. Fodor and Pylyshyn 1981, pp. 176–177.

45. Fodor and Pylyshyn 1981, p. 177.

reproduce items in space and may instantiate particulars, but they do not (uncontroversially) involve predication—one of the hallmarks of linguistic representation.[46] To show that the markers in a map that stand for elements in the environment—for example, squares—behave like subjects or like predicates would require additional arguments. For one thing, taking away a marker from a map does not leave us with a meaningless map in the same way in which taking away a subject from a sentence leaves us with a meaningless sentence. Thus, the simple consideration that percepts display the systematicity that comes from map-like representations is not sufficient to also show that linguistic representations are involved in perception.

Perhaps, we should think that perceptual systematicity is the ability to see, in analogous ways, different scenes that have common elements. Our capacity to see red and blue, and squares and triangles, allows us to see red squares and blue triangles, but also to see red triangles and blue squares. In this sense as well, vision is systematic, as some basic perceptual competences make sense of why we are able to see scenes that have common constituents.

How this perceptual ability is achieved has come to be known as the 'binding problem.'[47] There are different types of perceptual binding—for example, part, temporal, and location—but one important type consists of the capacity to bind together properties—such as shape and color—that are processed in specialized and sometimes separate visual areas. In giving a story of binding, we need a sense of how the visual system, having neurons that selectively respond to, say, red, blue, triangle, and square, binds them in different ways in different contexts. But although we may see this ability as a type of systematicity, this is not an ability achieved by recombining linguistic representations.

Notice first, that this preliminary rendition of binding seems to presume that there are dedicated channels for the detection of different colors and different shapes. We can be skeptical of this presumption on predictive coding grounds. As already mentioned in previous chapters, one of the insights of predictive coding accounts is that neurons in early visual areas lack fixed receptive fields.

46. Fodor and Pylyshyn 1988. See Rescorla 2009b for some relevant differences between the role of markers in a map and predicates.

47. Von der Malsburg 1995, Treisman 1996. See also O'Callaghan forthcoming for a multimodal perspective on binding.

Further, even if we concede that different elements need to be bound in perception, it is not clear that this ability requires linguistically structured representations. Accounts of binding typically appeal either to the role of selective attention—as features that are attended are processed as belonging together—or to signal-synchrony where groups of cells are bound to each other by their synchronized activation.[48] But, if this is true, then computations over map-like, or list-like representations seem sufficient to account for binding. We can think of signal synchrony or attention as what 'holds together' the features in a list. As Fodor and Pylyshyn concede, "lists, qua lists, have no [genuine linguistic] structure; any collection of items is a possible list."[49]

As in the case of productivity, the perceptual systematicity that we find in binding is not a feature that shows that perception operates on sensory and perceptual states that have linguistic format. Basic sensory abilities—for example, the ability to respond to shape and color—are bound together by attention and by concomitant activation. They are not bound together by predication.

The general difficulty, in this context, is that that productivity and systematicity are notions borrowed from linguistic analysis. Languages tend to be productive and systematic. We are in principle able to produce infinitely many new sentences, and the ability to understand certain sentences is intrinsically related to the ability to understand certain others. It is not clear, however, how to transfer these facts to perceptual and non linguistic states. It could, of course, be that perception displays the same basic structure and architecture of language—and that it issues representations with linguistic form—but showing that this is the case would require a lot more work.

The need for additional arguments may be less pressing in the case of thought because it is somewhat intuitive that thought has language-like form. The thought 'Chase loves Julio' seems to come in linguistic form, to involve predication and to have syntactic parts that are detachable. This same intuition, however, is not warranted in the case of perception. Whether perception has linguistic form is a debated issue. While it is true that, in most cases, we can describe what we see with sentences and propositions, this reflects the structure of perceptual *judgment*, not of perception *per se*.[50]

---

48. Treisman and Schmidt 1982.

49. Fodor and Pylyshyn 1988, p. 34. Text in brackets added by author.

50. Thanks to an anonymous referee for raising this point.

If this is right, then the usual considerations for supporting classicism do not straightforwardly apply to the perceptual case. Vision may plausibly be carried out by connectionist and non-classical digital systems that produce representations with no linguistic format. This raises a very interesting question: the question of the relation between perceptual states on the one hand, and beliefs and thoughts on the other. If the latter have linguistic form while the former do not, we are owed a story of both how (if at all) they interact, and of what is responsible for the change in format when we move from a given perception to a corresponding perceptual judgment and to a perceptual belief. I leave these questions for a future project.

In this section, I showed that the arguments in favor of classical architectures as models of thinking, do not work for perception. We have little reason to suppose that classicism is the only game in town to understand vision. We can then adopt an embedded account of visual processing while also being open to the fact that the classical computational theory of mind is true of other psychological capacities. Since the embedded view is also compatible with computationalism (non-restrictively defined) we have one more reason to accept it.

5.4 Conclusion

This chapter concludes the argument in favor of the embedded view introduced in chapter 2. It does so by showing that EV is compatible with computationalism. This is true for two reasons: first, there are perfectly legitimate models of computation that do not describe them as regimented operations on symbols or representations. Second, denying that the visual system performs computations in the classical sense does not amount to rejecting the classical computational theory of mind in its entirety.

We can then sum up the case in favor of a noncognitive account of vision. The embedded view has been shown to be a plausible model on both theoretical and empirical grounds. It fits well with current models of vision in cognitive psychology and it accords with reflection on the notion of representation. It is more responsive to the evidence, and it is capable of explaining a number of central visual phenomena without appeal to representations. The additional fact that the embedded model is compatible with computationalism constitutes a reason to favor it for those who like computationalism. By putting vision in its natural place, we come to appreciate that it is not a cognitive process.

Bibliography

Abernethy, B. (1991). Visual search strategies and decision-making in sport. *International Journal of Sport Psychology*, 22:189–210.

Abernethy, B., Neil, R., and Koning, P. (1994). Visual-perceptual and cognitive differences between expert, intermediate and novice snooker players. *Applied Cognitive Psychology*, 8:185–210.

Ahluwalia, A. (1978). An intra-cultural investigation of susceptibility to 'perspective' and 'non-perspective' spatial illusions. *British Journal of Psychology*, 69(22): 233–241.

Akins, K. (1996). Of sensory systems and the 'aboutness' of mental states. *The Journal of Philosophy*, 93(7):337–372.

Austin, J. L., Strawson, P. F., and Cousin, D. R. "Symposium: Truth." *Proceedings of the Aristotelian Society, Supplementary Volumes*, (1950):111–172.

Aydede, M. and Robbins, P. (2009). *The Cambridge handbook of situated cognition*. Cambridge University Press, New York.

Baillargeon, R. (1993). The object concept revisited: New directions in the investigation of infants' physical knowledge. In *Visual perception and cognition in infancy*, edited by C. Granud. Erlbaum, Hillsdale, NJ.

Bakin, J., Nakayama, K., and Gilbert, C. (2000). Visual responses in monkey areas V1 and V2 to three-dimensional surface configuration. *Journal of Neuroscience*, 20:8188–8198.

Ballard, D. H. (1991). Animate vision. *Artificial Intelligence*, 48(1):57–86.

Barlow, H. (1995). The neuron doctrine in perception. In *The cognitive neurosciences*, edited by M. Gazzaniga, pp. 415–435. MIT Press, Cambridge, MA.

Barrick, C., Taylor, D., and Correa, E. (2002). Color sensitivity and mood disorders: biology or metaphor? *Journal of Affective Disorder* 68:67–71.

Bechtel, W. (1993). The case for connectionism. *Philosophical Studies*, 71:119–154.

Bechtel, W. (1998). Representations and cognitive explanations: assessing the dynamicists challenge in cognitive science. *Cognitive Science*, 22(3):295–318.

Beer, R. (1995). A dynamical systems perspective on agent-environment interaction. *Artificial Intelligence*, 72:173–215.

Bennett, M. R. Hacker, P. M. (2003). *Philosophical foundations of neuroscience*. Blackwell, Oxford.

Bialystok, E. (2001). *Bilingualism in development: language, literacy, and cognition*. Cambridge University Press, Cambridge, UK.

Bialystok, E. and Martin, M. (2004). Attention and inhibition in bilingual children: Evidence from the dimensional change card sort task. *Developmental Science*, 7:325–339.

Bialystok, E. and Shapero, D. (2005). Ambiguous benefits: the effect of bilingualism on reversing ambiguous figures. *Developmental Science*, 8(6):595–604.

Biederman, I. and Shiffrar, M. (1987). Sexing day-old chicks: a case study and expert systems analysis of a difficult perceptual-learning task. *Journal of Experimental Psychology: Learning, Memory and Cognition*, 13(4):640–645.

Blakemore, R. and Frankel, R. (1981). Magnetic navigation in bacteria. *Scientific American*, 245(6):58–65.

Boghossian, P. (2008). Epistemic rules. *Journal of Philosophy*, 9:472–500 [Special issue: Epistemic Norms].

Boghossian, P. (2012). What is inference? *Philosophical Studies*. Article first published http://link.springer.com/article/10.1007%2Fs11098-012-9903-x

Boster, J. (1986). Exchange of varieties and information between aguarana manioc cultivators. *American Anthropologist*, 88:428–436.

Bozzi, P. (1980). Immagini consecutive e completamento amodale. In *Reports from the Institute of Psychology*. University of Trieste, Trieste, Italy.

Brainard, D. H. (2009). Bayesian approaches to color vision. *The visual neurosciences*, 4. Available online at <http://color.psych.upenn.edu/brainard/papers/BayesColorReview.pdf>.

Brentano, F. ([1874]2009). *Psychology from an empirical standpoint*. Routledge, Taylor and Francis.

Brewer, B. (2007). How to account for illusion. In *Disjunctivism: perception, action, knowledge*. edited by F. Macpherson and A. Haddock, A., pp. 168–180. Oxford University Press, Oxford.

Britz, J., Pitts, M., and Michel, C. (2009). Right parietal brain activity precedes perceptual alternation of bistable stimuli. *Cerebral Cortex*, 19:55–65.

Brogaard, B. (2011). Conscious vision for action versus unconscious vision for action? *Cognitive Science*, 35(6):1076–1104.

Brooks, R. (1991). Intelligence without representation. *Artificial Intelligence*, 47: 139–159.

Bruner, J. and Goodman, C. (1947). Value and need as organizing factors in perception. *Journal of Abnormal and Social Psychology*, 42(1):33–44.

Budd, M. (1987). Wittgenstein on seeing aspects. *Mind*, 96(381):1–17.

Burge, T. (1979). Individualism and the mental. In *Midwest Studies in Philosophy IV*, edited by P. A. French, T. E. Uehling, and H. K. Wettstein, pp. 73–121. University of Minnesota Press, Minneapolis.

Burge, T. (2008). Disjunctivism and perceptual psychology. *Philosophical Topics*, 33(1):1–78.

Burge, T. (2009). Perceptual objectivity. *Philosophical Review*, 118(3):285–324.

Burge, T. (2010). *Origins of objectivity*. Oxford University Press, Oxford.

Burge, T. (2011). Disjunctivism again. *Philosophical Explorations*, 14(1):43–80.

Campbell, J. (2002). *Reference and consciousness*. Clarendon Press, Oxford.

Cantwell-Smith, B. (1996). *On the origin of objects* (vol. 708). MIT Press, Cambridge, MA.

Carter, L. F. and Schooler, K. (1949). Value, need, and other factors in perception. *Psychological Review*, 56(4):200.

Chalmers, D. J. (1992). Syntactic transformations on distributed representations. In *Connectionist natural language processing*, pp. 46–55. Springer, New York.

Chalmers, D. (1993). Connectionism and compositionality: why Fodor and Pylyshyn were wrong. *Philosophical Psychology*, 6(3):305–320.

Chalmers, D. J. (2011). A computational foundation for the study of cognition. *Journal of Cognitive Science*, 12(4):323–357.

Chase, W. and Simon, H. (1973). Perception in chess. *Cognitive Psychology*, 4:55–81.

Chastain, G. and Brunham, C. (1975). The first glimpse determines the perception of an ambiguous figure. *Perception and Psychophysics*, 17(3):221–224.

Chemero, A. (2003). An outline of a theory of affordances. *Ecological psychology*, 15(2):181–195.

Chemero, A. (2009). *Radical embodied cognitive science*. MIT Press, Cambridge, MA.

Chomsky, N. (1959). A review of bf Skinner's verbal behavior. In Jakobovits, L. and Miron, M., editors, *Language*, 35(1):26–58.

Chomsky, N. (1980). Rules and representations. *The Behavioral and Brain Sciences*, 3:1–15.

Churchland, P. (1979). *Scientific realism and the plasticity of mind*. Cambridge University Press.

Churchland, P. (1981). Eliminative materialism and the propositional attitudes. *Journal of Philosophy*, 78:67–90.

Churchland, P. (1989). Perceptual plasticity and theoretical neutrality: a reply to Jerry Fodor. In *A neurocomputational perspective: The nature of mind and the structure of science*, pp. 255–280. MIT Press, Cambridge, MA.

Churchland, P. (1990). Cognitive activity in artificial neural networks. In *Thinking: An invitation to cognitive science*, edited by D. Osherson and E. Smith, pp. 372–381. MIT Press, Cambridge, MA.

Churchland, P. S. and Churchland, P. M. (1983). Stalking the wild epistemic engine. *A.P.A. Western Division Meetings*, 71(1):5–18.

Clark, A. (1997). *Being there: putting brain, body, and world together again*. MIT Press, Cambridge, MA.

Clark, A. (2001). Visual experience and motor action: are the bonds too tight? *Philosophical Review*, 110(4):495–519.

Clark, A. (2012). Whatever next? predictive brains, situated agents, and the future of cognitive science. *Behavioral and Brain Science*, pages 1–86.

Clark, A. and Chalmers, D. (1998). The extended mind. *Analysis*, 58:10–23.

Clark, A. and Grush, R. (1999). Towards a cognitive robotics. *Adaptive Behavior*, 7(1):5–16.

Clark, A. and Toribio, J. (1994). Doing without representing? *Synthese*, 101: 401–431.

Coren, S. and Girgus, J. (1972). Differentiation and decrement in the Müller-Lyer illusion. *Perception and Psychophysics*, 12(3):446–470.

Coren, S., Ward, L., and Enns, J. (1999). *Sensation and perception*. Harcourt College Publishing, Ft. Worth, TX.

Cowie, F. (1999). *What's within?: nativism reconsidered*. Oxford University Press, Oxford.

Cummins, R. (1983). *The nature of psychological explanation*. MIT Press Cambridge, MA.

Cummins, R. and Poirier, P. (2004). Representation and indication. *Representation in mind: new approaches to mental representation*, pp. 21–40, Elsevier, London.

Davies, M. (1987). Tacit knowledge and semantic theory: can a five per cent difference matter? *Mind*, 96(384):441–462.

De Groot, A. (1994). *Thought and choice in chess*. The Hague, The Netherlands.

Dennett, D. (1982). Styles of mental representation. *JSTOR: Proceedings of the Aristotelian Society*, 83:213–226.

Dennett, D. (1987). *The intentional stance*. MIT Press, Cambridge, MA.

Dennett, D. (1991). Real patterns. *The Journal of Philosophy*, 88(1):27–51.

Dennett, D. (1992). 'Filling in' versus finding out: a ubiquitous confusion in cognitive science. In *Cognition, conception, and methodological issues*, H. L. Pick., Jr. and P. Van Den Broek, authors, and D. C. Knill, editor, pp. 33–49. American Psychological Association, Washington, DC.

Deroy, O. (2013). Object-sensitivity versus cognitive penetrability of perception. *Philosophical Studies*, 162(1):87–107.

Deruelle, C., Barbet, I., Depy, D., and Fagot, J. (2000). Perception of partially occluded figures by baboons (papio papio). *Perception*, 29:1483–1497.

Descartes, R. ([1641] 1996). *Descartes: meditations on first philosophy: with selections from the objections and replies*. Cambridge University Press.

Desimone, R. and Duncan, J. (1995). Neural mechanisms of selective visual attention. *Annual Review of Neuroscience*, 18(1):193–222.

Diamond, A. (2002). Normal development of pre-frontal cortex from birth to young adulthood: cognitive functions, anatomy, and biochemistry. In *Principles of frontal lobe functioning*, edited by D. Stuss and R. Knight, pp. 466–503. Oxford University Press, New York.

Dretske, F. (1969). *Seeing and knowing*. University of Chicago Press, Chicago.

Dretske, F. (1981). *Knowledge and the flow of information*. MIT Press, Cambridge, MA.

Dretske, F. (1991). *Explaining behavior: reasons in a world of causes*. MIT Press, Cambridge, MA.

Dretske, F. (1997). *Naturalizing the mind*. MIT Press, Cambridge, MA.

Dretske, F. (2006). Perception without awareness. In *Perceptual experience*, edited by T. Gendler and J. Hawthorne, pp. 147–180. Clarendon Press, Oxford.

Dreyfus, H. L. (2002). Intelligence without representation–Merleau-Ponty's critique of mental representation the relevance of phenomenology to scientific explanation. *Phenomenology and the Cognitive Sciences*, 1(4):367–383.

Eberhardt, J. L., Goff, P. A., Purdie, V. J., Davies, P. G., et al. (2004). Seeing black: race, crime, and visual processing. *Journal of Personality and Social Psychology*, 87:876–893.

Eliasmith, C. (2007). How to build a brain: from function to implementation. *Synthese*, 159(3):373–388.

Elliffe, M. (1999). Performance measurement based on usable information. In *Information theory and the brain*, R. Baddeley, P. Hancock, and P. Foldiak, pp. 180–200. Cambridge University Press, Cambridge, UK.

Epstein, W., Park, J., and Casey, A. (1961). The current status of the size-distance hypotheses. *Psychological Bulletin*, 58(6):491–514.

Evans, G. (1981). Semantic theory and tacit knowledge. *Wittgenstein: to follow a rule*, edited by S. Holtzman and C. Leich, pp. 118–137. Routledge, London.

Evans, G. L. (1982). *The varieties of reference*. Oxford University Press on Demand.

Fagot, J., Barbet, I., Parron, C., and Deruelle, C. (2006). Amodal completion by baboons (papio papio): contribution of background depth cues. *Primates*, 47(2):145–150.

Fahle, M. and Morgan, M. (1996). No transfer of perceptual learning between similar stimuli in the same retinal position. *Current Biology*, 6(3):292–297.

Fineman, M. B. and Carlson, J. (1996). A comparison of the ponzo illusion with a textural analogue. *Perception & Psychophysics*, 14(1):31–33.

Firestone, C. and Scholl, B. J. (forthcoming). 'Top-down' effects where none should be found: tyhe el Greco fallacy in perception research. *Psychological Science*.

Fodor, J. (1975). *The language of thought*. Harvard University Press, Cambridge, MA.

Fodor, J. A. (1983). *Modularity of mind*. MIT Press, Cambridge, MA and London.

Fodor, J. A. (1984). Observation reconsidered. *Philosophy of Science*, 51(1):23–43.

Fodor, J. A. (1987a). *Psychosemantics*. MIT Press, Cambridge, MA.

Fodor, J. A. (1987b). Why paramecia don't have mental representations. *Midwest Studies in Philosophy*, 10(1):3–23.

Fodor, J. A. (1988). A reply to Churchland's 'perceptual plasticity and theoretical neutrality.' *Philosophy of Science*, 55(2):188–198.

Fodor, J. A. (1990a). *A theory of content and other essays*. MIT Press, Cambridge, MA.

Fodor, J. A. (1990b). Information and representation. *Information, language, and cognition*, edited by P. P. Hanson, pp. 175–190. University of British Columbia Press, Vancouver.

Fodor, J. A. (1998). *Concepts: where cognitive science went wrong*. Oxford University Press, New York.

Fodor, J. A. and Pylyshyn, Z. W. (1981). How direct is visual perception? some reflections on gibson's 'ecological approach.' *Cognition*, 9:139–196.

Fodor, J. A. and Pylyshyn, Z. W. (1988). Connectionism and cognitive architecture: a critical analysis. *Cognition*, 28(1):3–71.

Frank, D. A. and Greenberg, M. E. (1994). Creb: a mediator of long-term memory from mollusks to mammals. *Cell*, 79(1):5.

Freeman, W. J. and Skarda, C. A. (1990). Representations: who needs them. In *Brain organization and memory cells, systems, and circuits*, edited by J. L. McGaugh, N. Weinberger, and G. Lynch, pp. 375–380. Oxford University Press, New York.

Fujita, K. (1997). Perception of the Ponzo illusion by rhesus monkeys, chimpanzees, and humans: similarity and difference in the three primate species. *Perception & Psychophysics*, 59(2):284–292.

Fujita, K. (2001). Perceptual completion in rhesus monkeys (macaca mulatta) and pigeons (columba livia). *Perception & Psychophysics*, 63(1):115–125.

Fujita, K., Blough, D. S., and Blough, P. M. (1991). Pigeons see the Ponzo illusion. *Animal Learning & Behavior*, 19(3):283–293.

Gallistel, C. R. (1990). *The organization of learning*. MIT Press, Cambridge, MA.

Ganson, T., Bronner, B., and Kerr, A. (2012). Burge's defense of perceptual content. *Philosophy and Phenomenological Research*. Article first published online. DOI: 10.1111/j.1933-1592.2012.00632.x © 2012 Philosophy and Phenomenological

Geisler, W. S. (2008). Visual perception and the statistical properties of natural scenes. *Annual Review of Psychology*, 59:167–192.

Geisler, W., Perry, J., Super, B., Gallogly, D., et al. (2001). Edge co-occurrence in natural images predicts contour grouping performance. *Vision Research*, 41(6):711–724.

Gerbino, W. and Zabai, C. (2003). The joint. *Acta Psychologica*, 114:331–353.

Gibson, J. (1966). *The senses considered as perceptual systems*. Houghton Mifflin, Boston.

Gibson, J. (1979). *The ecological approach to visual perception*. Houghton Mifflin, Boston.

Girgus, J. J., Rock, I., and Egatz, R. (1977). The effect of knowledge of reversibility on the reversibility of ambiguous figures. *Perception & Psychophysics*, 22(6):550–556.

Glen, J. (1940). Ocular movements in reversibility of perspective. *The Journal of General Psychology*, 23(2):243–281.

Goldstein, E. B. (2013). *Sensation and perception*. Cengage Learning, Stamford, CT.

Goldstone, R. L. (1998). Perceptual learning. *Annual Review of Psychology*, 49(1): 585–612.

Goldstone, R. L. (2003). Learning to perceive while perceiving to learn. In *Perceptual organization in vision: behavioral and neural perspectives*, edited by R. Kimchi, M. Behrmann, and C. Olson, pp. 233–278. Erlbaum, Hillsdale, NJ.

Gopnik, A. and Rosati, A. (2001). Duck or rabbit? Reversing ambiguous figures and understanding ambiguous representations. *Developmental Science*, 4(2): 175–183.

Gorman, R. P. and Sejnowski, T. J. (1988). Analysis of hidden units in a layered network trained to classify sonar targets. *Neural Networks*, 1(1): 75–89.

Gracheva, E. O., Ingolia, N. T., Kelly, Y. M., Cordero-Morales, J. F., et al. (2010). Molecular basis of infrared detection by snakes. *Nature*, 464(7291):1006–1011.

Gregory, R. L. (1963). Distortion of visual space as inappropriate constancy scaling. *Nature*, 199(678–91):1.

Gregory, R. (1970). *The intelligent eye*. McGrawy-Hill, New York.

Grice, H. P. (1957). Meaning. *The Philosphical Review*, 66(3):377–388.

Grosof, D., Shaplet, R., and Hawken, M., (1993). Macaque v1 neurons can signal 'illusory' contours. *Nature*, 365:550–552.

Grossberg, S. (1993). A solution of the figure-ground problem for biological vision. *Neural Networks*, 6(4):463–483.

Grush, R. (1997). The architecture of representation. *Philosophical Psychology*, 10(1):5–23.

Gunther, Y. H. (2003). (Ed.). *Essays on nonconceptual content*. MIT Press, Cambridge, MA.

Hamaguchi, K. (2001). An examination of the perspective theory on the Müller-Lyer illusion: in relation to the texture gradient. *Research Reports of Kochi University: Humanities*, 50:185–191.

Hansen, T., Olkkonen, M., Walter, S., and Gegenfurtner, K. R. (2006). Memory modulates color appearance. *Nature Neuroscience*, 9(11):1367–1368.

Hatfield, G. C. (2009). *Perception and cognition: essays in the philosophy of psychology*. Clarendon Press, Oxford.

Haugeland, J. (1998). Having thought: *essays in the metaphysics of mind*. Harvard University Press, Cambridge, MA.

Heft, H. (1989). Affordances and the body: an intentional analysis of Gibson's ecological approach to visual perception. *Journal for the Theory of Social Behaviour*, 19(1):1–30.

Hohwy, J. (2007). Functional integration and the mind. *Synthese*, 159(3):315–328.

Hohwy, J., Roepstorff, A., and Friston, K. (2008). Predictive coding explains binocular rivalry: an epistemological review. *Cognition*, 108(3):687–701.

Hosoya, T., Baccus, S. A., and Meister, M. (2005). Dynamic predictive coding by the retina. Nature, 436(7047):71–77.

Howe, C. and Purves, D. (2005a). The Müller-Lyer illusion explained by the statistics of image source relationships. *Proceedings of the National Academy of Sciences of the United States of America*, 102(4):1234–1239.

Howe, C. and Purves, D. (2005b). *Perceiving geometry: geometrical illusions explained by natural scene statistics.* Springer Science and Business Media, New York.

Howe, C. Q., Beau Lotto, R., and Purves, D. (2006). Comparison of Bayesian and empirical ranking approaches to visual perception. *Journal of Theo-retical Biology*, 241(4):866–875.

Howe, C., Yang, Z., and Purves, D. (2005). The Poggendorff illusion explained by natural scene geometry. *Proceedings of the National Academy of Science*, 102(21):7707–7712.

Hubel, D. H. and Wiesel, T. N. (1962). Receptive fields, binocular interaction and functional architecture in the cat's visual cortex. *The Journal of Physiology*, 160(1):106.

Hubel, D. H. and Wiesel, T. N. (1968). Receptive fields and functional architecture of monkey striate cortex. *The Journal of Physiology*, 195(1):215–243.

Hugenberg, K. and Bodenhausen, G. V. (2003). Facing prejudice implicit prejudice and the perception of facial threat. *Psychological Science*, 14(6): 640–643.

Hurley, S. L. (2002). *Consciousness in action.* Harvard University Press, Cambridge, MA.

Ito, J., Nikolaev, A. R., Luman, M., Aukes, M. F., et al. (2003). Perceptual switching, eye movements, and the bus paradox. *Perception-London*, 32(6):681–698.

James, W. ([1890]1983). *Principles of psychology.* Harvard University Press, Cambridge, MA.

Jastrow, J. (1899). The mind's eye. *Popular Science Monthly*, 54:299–312.

Jehee, J. F. and Ballard, D. H. (2009). Predictive feedback can account for biphasic responses in the lateral geniculate nucleus. *PLoS Computational Biology*, 5(5):e1000373.

Johnson, K. E. and Mervis, C. B. (1997). Effects of varying levels of expertise on the basic level of categorization. *Journal of Experimental Psychology: General*, 126(3):248.

Kanizsa, G. (1979). *Organization in vision: essays on Gestalt perception.* Praeger New York.

Kanizsa, G. (1985). Seeing and thinking. *Acta Psychologica*, 59(1):23–33.

Kanizsa, G. and Gerbino, W. (1982). Amodal completion: seeing or thinking. In *Organization and representation in perception*, edited by J. Beck, pp. 167–190. Erlbaum, Hillsdale, NJ.

Kardong, K. V. and Mackessy, S. P. (1991). The strike behavior of a congenitally blind rattlesnake. *Journal of Herpetology*, 25(2):208–211.

Karmiloff-Smith, A. (1986). From meta-processes to conscious access: evidence from children's metalinguistic and repair data. *Cognition*, 23(2):95–147.

Kleinschmidt, A., Büchel, C., Zeki, S., and Frackowiak, R. (1998). Human brain activity during spontaneously reversing perception of ambiguous figures. *Proceedings of the Royal Society of London. Series B: Biological Sciences*, 265(1413): 2427–2433.

Koffka, K. (1935). *Principles of Gestalt psychology*. Harcourt, Brace, New York.

Kripke, S. (1982). On rules and private language. In *The philosophy of language*, edited by A. P. Martinich, pp. 531–534. Oxford University Press, New York.

Kuhn, T. S. ([1962]2012). *The structure of scientific revolutions*. University of Chicago Press.

Kundel, H. L. and Nodine, C. F. (1975). Interpreting chest radiographs without visual search. *Radiology*, 116(3):527–532.

Leopold, D. A. and Logothetis, N. K. (1999). Multistable phenomena: changing views in perception. *Trends in Cognitive Sciences*, 3(7):254–264.

Lettvin, J. Y., Maturana, H. R., McCulloch, W. S., and Pitts, W. H. (1959). What the frog's eye tells the frog's brain. *Proceedings of the IRE*, 47(11):1940–1951.

Levin, D. T. and Banaji, M. R. (2006). Distortions in the perceived lightness of faces: the role of race categories. *Journal of Experimental Psychology General*, 135(4):501.

Long, F. and Purves, D. (2003). Natural scene statistics as the universal basis of color context effects. *Proceedings of the National Academy of Sciences*, 100(25): 15190–15193.

Lotto, R. B. and Purves, D. (2001). An empirical explanation of the chubb illusion. *Journal of Cognitive Neuroscience*, 13(5):547–555.

Lotto, R. B., Williams, S. M., and Purves, D. (1999). Mach bands as empirically derived associations. *Proceedings of the National Academy of Sciences*, 96(9): 5245–5250.

Lycan, W. (2006). Representational theories of consciousness. In *Stanford encyclopedia of philosophy*, edited by E. N. Zalta.

Lyons, J. (2011). Circularity, reliability, and the cognitive penetrability of perception. *Philosophical Issues*, 21(1):289–311.

Machery, E. (2009). *Doing without concepts*. Oxford University Press, Oxford.

Macpherson, F. (2012). Cognitive penetration of colour experience: rethinking the issue in light of an indirect mechanism. *Philosophy and Phenomenological Research*, 84(1):24–62.

Maloney, L. T., and Mamassian, P., (2009). Bayesian decision theory as a model of human visual perception: testing Bayesian transfer. *Visual neuroscience*, 26(01):147–155.

Malsburg, C. (1995). Binding in models of perception and brain function. *Current Opinion in Neurobiology*, 5(4):520–526.

Mamassian, P. and Landy, M. S. (1998). Observer biases in the 3d interpretation of line drawings. *Vision Research*, 38(18):2817–2832.

Mamassian, P., Landy, M. S., Maloney, L. T., Rao, R., et al. (2002). Bayesian modelling of visual perception. In *Probabilistic models of the brain: perception and neural function*, edited by R. P. N. Rao, B. A. Olshausen, and M. S. Lewicki, pp. 13–36. MIT Press,Cambridge, MA.

Mandelbaum, E. (unpublished). Attitude, inference, association: On the propositional structure of implicit bias. Available at <http://people.fas.harvard.edu/mandelbaum/Attitude>.

Mandik, P. (2005). Action-oriented representation. In *Cognition and the brain: the philosophy and neuroscience movement*, edited by K. Akins and A. Brooks, pp. 284–305. Cambridge University Press, Cambridge.

Margolis, E. and Laurence, S. (2007). The ontology of concepts—abstract objects or mental representations? 1. *Noûs*, 41(4):561–593.

Marr, D. (1982). *Vision: a computational investigation into the human representation and processing of visual information*. Henry Holt, New York.

Marr, D. and Hildreth, E. (1980). Theory of edge detection. *Proceedings of the Royal Society of London. Series B; Biological Sciences*, 207(1167):187–217.

Martin, M. G. (2004). The limits of self-awareness. *Philosophical Studies*, 120(1): 37–89.

Mather, G. (2009). *Foundations of sensation and perception* (vol. 2) Psychology Press, Philadelphia.

Matlin, M. W. and Foley, H. J. (1997). *Sensation and perception*. Allyn and Bacon, Boston, London.

Matthen, M. (2005). *Seeing, doing, and knowing: a philosophical theory of sense perception*. Clarendon Press, Oxford.

McClamrock, R. (1995). *Existential cognition: computational minds in the world*. University of Chicago Press.

McDowell, J. (1996). *Mind and world* (with a new introduction by the author). Harvard University Press, Cambridge, MA.

Michotte, A., Thinès, G., and Crabbé, G. (1964). *Les complements amodaux des structures perceptives*. Institut de Psychologie de l'Université de Louvain.

Millikan, R. G. (1989). Biosemantics. *The Journal of Philosophy*, 86(6):281–297.

Millikan, R. G. (1995). Pushmi-pullyu representations. *Philosophical Perspectives*, 9:185–200.

Milner, A. D. and Goodale, M. A. (1995). *The visual brain in action*. Oxford University Press, New York.

Mole, C. (2011). *Attention is cognitive unison: an essay in philosophical psychology*. Oxford University Press, New York.

Myles-Worsley, M., Johnston, W. A., and Simons, M. A. (1988). The influence of expertise on x-ray image processing. *Journal of Experimental Psychology: Learning, Memory, and Cognition*, 14(3):553.

Nagasaka, Y. and Osada, Y. (2000). Subjective contours, amodal completion, and transparency in animals. *Japanese Journal of Animal Psychology*, 50:61–73.

Nagasaka, Y. and Wasserman, E. A. (2008). Amodal completion of moving objects by pigeons. *Perception*, 37(4):557.

Nakamura, N., Fujita, K., Ushitani, T., Miyata, H., et al. (2006). Perception of the standard and the reversed Müller-Lyer figures in pigeons (columba livia) and humans (homo sapiens). *Journal of Comparative Psychology*, 120(3):252–260.

Nakatani, H. and van Leeuwen, C. (2006). Transient synchrony of distant brain areas and perceptual switching in ambiguous figures. *Biological Cybernetics*, 94(6):445–457.

Nanay, B. (2009). Shape constancy, not size constancy: a (partial) explanation for the Müller-Lyer illusion. In *Proceedings of the 31st Annual Conference of the Cognitive Science Society (CogSci 2009)*, pp. 579–584. Erlbaum, Hillsdale, NJ.

Noë, A. (2002). Is the visual world a grand illusion? *Journal of Consciousness Studies*, 9(5–6):1–12.

Noë, A. (2004). *Action in perception*. MIT Press, Cambridge, MA.

Noë, A. (2012). *Varieties of presence*. Harvard University Press, Cambridge, MA.

Norman, D. A. (1999). Affordance, conventions, and design. *Interactions*, 6(3): 38–43.

Norman, J. (2002). Two visual systems and two theories of perception: an attempt to reconcile the constructivist and ecological approaches. *Behavioral and Brain Sciences*, 25(1):73–96.

Nundy, S. and Purves, D. (2002). A probabilistic explanation of brightness scaling. *Proceedings of the National Academy of Sciences*, 99(22):14482–14487.

Obermayer, K., Sejnowski, T., and Blasdel, G. (1995). Neural pattern formation via a competitive hebbian mechanism. *Behavioural Brain Research*, 66(1):161–167.

O'Callaghan, C. (2007). *Sounds: a philosophical theory*. Oxford University Press.

O'Callaghan, C. (forthcoming). Intermodal binding awareness. In *Sensory integration and the unity of consciousness*, edited by D. Bennett and C. Hill. MIT Press, Cambridge, MA. Available online at <http://ocallaghan.rice.edu// research/papers/ocallaghan-201x- Binding.pdf>.

O'Regan, J. K., Noë, A., et al. (2001). A sensorimotor account of vision and visual consciousness. *Behavioral and Brain Sciences*, 24(5):939–972.

O'Reilly, R. C. and Munakata, Y. (2000). *Computational explorations in cognitive neuroscience: understanding the mind by simulating the brain*. MIT Press/Bradford Books, Cambridge, MA.

Orlandi, N. (2010). Are sensory properties represented in perceptual experience? *Philosophical Psychology*, 23(6):721–740.

Orlandi, N. (2011a). Ambiguous figures and representationalism. *Phenomenology and the Cognitive Sciences*, 10(3):307–323.

Orlandi, N. (2011b). Embedded seeing: vision in the natural world. *Nous*, 47(4): 727–747.

Orlandi, N. (2012a). Embedded seeing-as: multi-stable visual perception without interpretation. *Philosophical Psychology*, 25(4):555–573.

Orlandi, N. (2012b). Visual switching: the illusion of instantaneity and visual search. *Review of Philosophy and Psychology*, 3(4):469–480.

O'Toole, A. J. and Abdi, H. (1989). Connectionist approaches to visuallybased facial feature extraction. *Advances in Cognitive Science*, 2:123.

Palmer, S. E. (1999). *Vision science: photons to phenomenology* (vol. 1). MIT Press, Cambridge, MA.

Papert, S. (1961). Centrally produced geometrical illusions. *Nature*, 191:733.

Parks, T. E. and Rock, I. (2000). *Looking at looking: an introduction to the intelligence of vision*. Sage Publications, Thousand Oaks, CA.

Payne, B. K. (2006). Weapon bias split-second decisions and unintended stereotyping. *Current Directions in Psychological Science*, 15(6):287–291.

Payne, B. K. (2001). Prejudice and perception: the role of automatic and controlled processes in misperceiving a weapon. *Journal of Personality and Social Psychology*, 81(2):181–192.

Payne, B. K. (2006). Weapon bias split-second decisions and unintended stereotyping. *Current Directions in Psychological Science*, 15(6):287–291.

Peacocke, C. (1992). *A study of concepts*. MIT Press, Cambridge, MA.

Perrett, D., Hietanen, J., Oram, M., Benson, P., et al. (1992). Organization and functions of cells responsive to faces in the temporal cortex [and discussion]. *Philosophical Transactions of the Royal Society of London. Series B: Biological Sciences*, 335(1273):23–30.

Pessoa, L., Thompson, E., and Noë, A. (1998). Finding out about filling-in: a guide to perceptual completion for visual science and the philosophy of perception. *Behavioral and Brain Sciences*, 21(6):723–748.

Piaget, J. ([1999]1954). *The construction of reality in the child* (vol. 20). Psychology Press, Hove, East Sussex, UK.

Piccinini, G. (2004). Functionalism, computationalism, and mental states. *Studies in History and Philosophy of Science Part A*, 35(4):811–833.

Piccinini, G. (2007). Computing mechanisms*. *Philosophy of Science*, 74(4):501–526.

Piccinini, G. (2008a). Computation without representation. *Philosophical Studies*, 137(2):205–241.

Piccinini, G. (2008b). Computers. *Pacific Philosophical Quarterly*, 89:32–73.

Piccinini, G. (2009). Computationalism in the philosophy of mind. *Philosophy Compass*, 4(3):515–532.

Piccinini, G. (2011). Computationalism. In *Oxford handbook of philosophy and cognitive science*, edited by E. Margolis, R. Samuels, and S. P. Stich, pp. 222–249. Oxford University Press.

Piccinini, G. and Bahar, S. (2012). Neural computation and the computational theory of cognition. *Cognitive Science*, 34:453–488.

Piccinini, G. and Scarantino, A. (2011). Information processing, computation, and cognition. *Journal of Biological Physics*, 37(1):1–38.

Plebe, A. and Domenella, R. G. (2007). Object recognition by artificial cortical maps. *Neural Networks*, 20(7):763–780.

Poggio, T. and Edelman, S. (1990). A network that learns to recognize 3d objects. *Nature*, 343(6255):263–266.

Poggio, T., Fahle, M., and Edelman, S. (1992). Fast perceptual learning in visual hyperacuity. *Science*, 256(5059):1018–1021.

Posner, M. I. and Petersen, S. E. (1990). The attention system of the human brain. *Annual Review of Neuroscience*, 13:25–42.

Price, H. H. (1950). *Perception*. Metheun, London.

Prinz, J. (2000). The ins and outs of consciousness. *Brain and Mind*, 1(2):245–256.

Prinz, J. J. (2012). *The conscious brain*. Oxford University Press, New York.

Purves, D. and Lotto, R. B. (2003). *Why we see what we do: an empirical theory of vision*. Sinauer Associates, Sunderland, MA.

Purves, D. and Lotto, R. B. (2011). Why we see what we do redux: An empirical theory of vision. Sinauer Associates.

Purves, D., Shimpi, A., and Lotto, R. B. (1999). An empirical explanation of the cornsweet effect. *The Journal of Neuroscience*, 19(19):8542–8551.

Putnam, H. (1973). Meaning and reference. *The Journal of Philosophy*, 70(19): 699–711.

Putnam, H. (1988). *Representation and reality* (vol. 454). Cambridge University Press.

Pylyshyn, Z. (1984). *Computation and cognition*. Cambridge University Press.

Pylyshyn, Z. (1999). Is vision continuous with cognition? the case for cognitive impenetrability of visual perception. *Behavioral and Brain Sciences*, 22(3):341–365.

Pylyshyn, Z. (2009). Perception, representation, and the world: the finst that binds. In *Computation, cognition, and Pylyshyn*, edited by D. Dedrick and L. Trick, pp. 3–48. MIT Press, Cambridge, MA. Available online at <ruccs.rutgers.edu/faculty/pylyshyn/Dedrick&TrickFinal.pdf>.

Rae, R. and Ritter, H. J. (1998). Recognition of human head orientation based on artificial neural networks. *IEEE Transactions on Neural Networks*, 9(2):257–265.

Ramachandran, V. S. (1988). Perceiving shape from shading. *Scientific American*, 259(2):76–83.

Ramsey, W. (1997). Do connectionist representations earn their explanatory keep? *Mind & Language*, 12(1):34–66.

Ramsey, W. M. (2007). *Representation reconsidered*. Cambridge University Press.

Ramsey, W., Stich, S., and Garon, J. (1991). Connectionism, eliminativism, and the future of folk psychology. In *Philosophy and connectionist theory*, edited by W. Ramsey, D. E. Rumelhart, and S. P. Stich, pp. 199–228. Erlbaum, Hillsdale, NJ.

Rao, R. P. and Sejnowski, T. J. (2002). Predictive coding, cortical feedback, and spike-timing dependent plasticity. In *Probabilistic models of the brain: perception and neural function*, edited by R. P. N. Rao, B. A. Olshauser, and M. S. Lewicki, p. 297. MIT Press, Cambridge, MA.

Recanati, F. (2002). Does linguistic communication rest on inference? *Mind & Language*, 17(1-2):105–126.

Rescorla, M. (2009a). Cognitive maps and the language of thought. *The British Journal for the Philosophy of Science*, 60(2):377–407.

Rescorla, M. (2009b). Predication and cartographic representation. *Synthese*, 169(1):175–200.

Rescorla, M. (2012). How to integrate representation into computational modeling, and why we should. *Journal of Cognitive Science*, 13(1):1–38.

Rescorla, M. (2014). The causal relevance of content to computation. *Philosophy and Phenomenological Research*, 88(1):173–208.

Rescorla, M. (forthcoming). Bayesian perceptual psychology. In *The Oxford handbook of the philosophy of perception*, edited by M. Matthen. Oxford University Press.

Ricci, C. and Blundo, C. (1990). Perception of ambiguous figures after focal brain lesions. *Neuropsychologia*, 28(11):1163–1173.

Rock, I. (1983). *The logic of perception*. MIT Press, Cambridge, MA.

Rock, I. (1997). *Indirect perception*. MIT Press, Cambridge, MA.

Rock, I. and Anson, R. (1979). Illusory contours as the solution to a problem. *Perception*, 8:665–681.

Rock, I., Gopnik, A., and Hall, S. (1994). Do young children reverse ambiguous figures? *Perception-London*, 23:635–635.

Rock, I. Mitchener, K. (1992). Further evidence of failure of reversal of ambiguous figures by uninformed subjects. *Perception*, 21(1):39–45.

Ropar, D., Mitchell, P., and Ackroyd, K. (2003). Do children with autism find it difficult to offer alternative interpretations to ambiguous figures? *British Journal of Developmental Psychology*, 21(3):387–395.

Rosch, E., Mervis, C. B., Gray, W. D., Johnson, D. M., et al. (1976). Basic objects in natural categories. *Cognitive Psychology*, 8(3):382–439.

Rosenblum, M., Yacoob, Y., and Davis, L. S. (1996). Human expression recognition from motion using a radial basis function network architecture. *IEEE Transactions on Neural Networks*, 7(5):1121–1138.

Rowlands, M. (1999). *The body in mind: understanding cognitive processes*. Cambridge University Press.

Rowlands, M. (2006). *Body language: representation in action*. MIT Press/Bradford Books, Cambridge, MA.

Rupert, R. D. (2004). Challenges to the hypothesis of extended cognition. *The Journal of Philosophy*, 101(8):389–428.

Ryle, G. (1949). *The concept of mind*. University of Chicago Press.

Sabisch, T., Ferguson, A., and Bolouri, H. (2000). Identification of complex shapes using a self organizing neural system. *IEEE Transactions on Neural Networks*, 11(4):921–934.

Sabo, D. (unpublished). Between empiricism and rationalism: The case of the sensory concepts. Unpublished manuscript available upon request.

Sabo, D. (2013). Where Concepts Come from: Learning Concepts by Description and by Demonstration. *Erkenntnis*, (2013):1–19.

Sanford, R. N. (1936). The effects of abstinence from food upon imaginal processes: a preliminary experiment. *The Journal of Psychology*, 2(1):129–136.

Sato, A., Kanazawa, S., and Fujita, K. (1997). Perception of object unity in a chimpanzee (pan troglodytes). *Japanese Psychological Research*, 39(3):191–199.

Scarantino, A. (2003). Affordances explained. *Philosophy of Science*, 70(5):949–961.

Schacter, D. L. (1987). Implicit memory: history and current status. *Journal of Experimental Psychology: Learning, Memory, and Cognition*, 13(3):501.

Schellenberg, S. (2010). The particularity and phenomenology of perceptual experience. *Philosophical Studies*, 149(1):19–48.

Schellenberg, S. (2011). Perceptual content defended. *Noûs*, 45(4):714–750.

Searle, J. R. (1980). Minds, brains, and programs. *Behavioral and Brain Sciences*, 3(3):417–457.

Segal, G. (1989). Seeing what is not there. *The Philosophical Review*, 98(2): 189–214.

Sejnowski, T. J. and Rosenberg, C. R. (1987). Parallel networks that learn to pronounce english text. *Complex Systems*, 1(1):145–168.

Sekuler, A. B., Lee, J. A., Shettleworth, S. J., et al. (1996). Pigeons do not complete partly occluded figures. *Perception-London*, 25:1909–1909.

Sekuler, A. B. and Palmer, S. E. (1992). Perception of partly occluded objects: a microgenetic analysis. *Journal of Experimental Psychology: General*, 121(1):95.

Sellars, W. (1954). Some reflections on language games. *Philosophy of Science*, 21(3):204–228.

Shannon, C. E. and Weaver, W. (1948). A mathematical theory of communication. *The Bell System Technical Journal*, 27:379–423.

Shapiro, Lawrence A. (1993). "Content, kinds, and individualism in Marr's theory of vision." *The Philosophical Review*, 102.4:489–513.

Shi, Y. Q. and Sun, H. (1999). *Image and video compression for multimedia engineering: fundamentals, algorithms, and standards*. CRC Press, Boca Raton, FL.

Siegel, S. (2006). Which properties are represented in perception. In *Perceptual experience*, edited by T. S. Gendler and J. Hawthorne, pp. 481–503. Oxford University Press.

Siegel, S. (2009). The visual experience of causation. *The Philosophical Quarterly*, 59(236):519–540.

Siegel, S. (2010). *The contents of visual experience*. Oxford University Press.

Siegel, S. (2012). Cognitive penetrability and perceptual justification. *Nous*, 46(2):201–222.

Siegel, S. (2013). Can selection effects on experience influence its rational role. *Oxford Studies in Epistemology*, 4.

Siewert, C. P. (1998). *The significance of consciousness*. Princeton University Press, Princeton, NJ.

Simon, H. A. and Barenfeld, M. (1969). Information processing analysis of perceptual processes in problem solving. *Psychological Review*, 76(5):473–483.

Simons, D. J. and Rensink, R. A. (2005). Change blindness: past, present, and future. *Trends in Cognitive Sciences*, 9(1):16–20.

Sloman, S. A. (1996). The empirical case for two systems of reasoning. *Psychological Bulletin*, 119(1):3.

Slotnick, S. D. and Yantis, S. (2005). Common neural substrates for the control and effects of visual attention and perceptual bistability. *Cognitive Brain Research*, 24(1):97–108.

Smith, E. R. and DeCoster, J. (1999). Associative and rule based processing. In *Dual-process theories in social psychology*, edited by S. Chaiken and Y, Trope, pp. 323–336. Guilford Press, New York.

Smolensky, P. (1988a). The constituent structure of connectionist mental states: a reply to Fodor and Pylyshyn. *The Southern Journal of Philosophy*, 26(S1): 137–161.

Smolensky, P. (1988b). On the proper treatment of connectionism. *Behavioral and Brain Sciences*, 11(1):1–74.

Spelke, E. S. (1990). Principles of object perception. *Cognitive Science*, 14(1):29–56.

Sperber, D. and Wilson, D. (1987). Précis of relevance: communication and cognition. *Behavioral and Brain Sciences*, 10(04):697–710.

Stanikunas, R., Vaitkevicius, H., and Kulikowski, J. J. (2004). Investigation of color constancy with a neural network. *Neural Networks*, 17(3):327–337.

Stanley, J. (2011). *Know how*. Oxford University Press, Oxford.

Sterman, J. D. (1994). Learning in and about complex systems. *System Dynamics Review*, 10(2–3):291–330.

Sterzer, P. and Kleinschmidt, A. (2007). A neural basis for inference in perceptual ambiguity. *Proceedings of the National Academy of Sciences*, 104(1):323–328.

Stewart, B. D. (2007). *Bringing automatic stereotyping under control: implementation Iintentions as Efficient means of thought control*. The Ohio State University.

Stich, S. and Nichols, S. (1992). Folk psychology: simulation or tacit theory? *Mind & Language*, 7(1-2):35–71.

Stich, S. P. (1983). *From folk psychology to cognitive science: the case against belief.* MIT Press, Cambridge, MA.

Stoffregen, T. A. (2003). Affordances as properties of the animal-environment system. *Ecological Psychology*, 15(2):115–134.

Stokes, D. (2012). Perceiving and desiring: a new look at the cognitive penetrability of experience. *Philosophical Studies*, 158(3):477–492.

Stone, J. V. (2011). Footprints sticking out of the sand (part ii): children's Bayesian priors for shape and lighting direction. Perception, 40(2):175–190.

Stone, J. V. and Pascalis, O. (2010). Footprints sticking out of the sand (part i): children's perception of naturalistic and embossed symbol stimuli. Perception, 39(9):1254–1260.

Stratton, G. M. (1896). Some preliminary experiments on vision without inversion of the retinal image. *Psychological Review*, 3(6):611–617.

Sugita, Y. (1999). Grouping of image fragments in primary visual cortex. *Nature*, 401(6750):269–272.

Thompson, E. (2007). *Mind in life: biology, phenomenology, and the sciences of mind*. Belknap Press, Cambridge, MA.

Tong, F., Meng, M., and Blake, R. (2006). Neural bases of binocular rivalry. *Trends in Cognitive Sciences*, 10(11):502–511.

Toppino, T. C. (2003). Reversible-figure perception: mechanisms of intentional control. *Perception & Psychophysics*, 65(8):1285–1295.

Travis, C. (2004). The silence of the senses. *Mind*, 113(449):57–94.

Treisman, A. (1996). The binding problem. *Current Opinion in Neurobiology*, 6(2):171–178.

Treisman, A. and Schmidt, H. (1982). Illusory conjunctions in the perception of objects. *Cognitive psychology*, 14(1):107–141.

Turvey, M. (1992). Affordances and prospective control: an outline of the ontology. *Ecological Psychology*, 4(3):173–187.

Tye, M. (1997). *Ten problems of consciousness: a representational theory of the phenomenal mind*. MIT Press, Cambridge, MA.

Ullman, S. (1979). *The interpretation of visual motion* (vol. 28). MIT Press, Cambridge, MA.

Ullman, S. (1980). *Against direct perception*. Cambridge University Press.

Ushitani, T. and Fujita, K. (2005). Pigeons do not perceptually complete partly occluded photos of food: An ecological approach to the 'pigeon problem.' *Behavioural Processes*, 69:67–78.

Van Gelder, T. (1990). Compositionality: a connectionist variation on a classical theme. *Cognitive Science*, 14(3):355–384.

Van Gelder, T. (1995). What might cognition be, if not computation? *The Journal of Philosophy*, 92(7):345–381.

Vetter, G., Haynes, J., and Pfaff, S. (2000). Evidence for multistability in the visual perception of pigeons. *Vision Research*, 40(16):2177–2186.

Von Békésy, G. (1967). *Sensory inhibition*. Princeton University Press, Princeton, NJ.

Von der Heydt, R., Peterhans, E., and Baumgartner, G. (1984). Illusory contours and cortical neuron responses. *Science*, 224(4654):1260–1262.

Von Helmholtz, H. (1924 (2005)). *Treatise on physiological optics* (vol. 3). Dover Publications, New York.

Vrins, S., de Wit, T. C., van Lier, R., et al. (2009). Bricks, butter, and slices of cucumber: investigating semantic influences in amodal completion. *Perception*, 38(1):17–29.

Wagemans, J., Elder, J. H., Kubovy, M., Palmer, S. E., et al. (2012). A century of Gestalt psychology in visual perception: I. perceptual grouping and figure–ground organization. *Psychological Bulletin*, 138(6):1218–1252.

Wallach, H. (1948). Brightness constancy and the nature of achromatic colors. *Journal of Experimental Psychology*, 38(3):310.

Weidner, R. and Fink, G. R. (2007). The neural mechanisms underlying the Müller-Lyer illusion and its interaction with visuospatial judgments. *Cerebral Cortex*, 17(4):878–884.

Weiskopf, D. A. (2008). The origins of concepts. *Philosophical Studies*, 140(3): 359–384.

Wertheimer, M. (1923(1938)). Laws of organization in perceptual forms. In *A source book of Gestalt psychology*, edited by W. D. Ellis, pp. 71–88. Gestalt Journal Press, Gouldsboro, ME.

Wilson, R. A. (2004). *Boundaries of the mind: the individual in the fragile sciences-cognition*. Cambridge University Press.

Wilson, R. A. (2010). Extended vision. In *Perception, action and consciousness*, edited by N. Gangopadhyay, M. Madary, & F. Spicer, pp. 277–290. Oxford University Press.

Wittgenstein, L. ([1953]2010). *Philosophical investigations*. Wiley-Blackwell.

Wollheim, R. (1980). *Art and its objects*. Cambridge University Press, Cambridge, UK.

Xu, F., Carey, S. (1996). Infants metaphysics: the case of numerical identity. *Cognitive Psychology*, 30(2):111–153.

Xu, F., Carey, S., and Quint, N. (2004). The emergence of kind-based object individuation in infancy. *Cognitive Psychology*, 49(2):155.

Yanagisawa, N. (1939). An experimental study on a modified Müller-Lyer figure (1). *Japanese Journal of Psychology*, 14:321–326.

Yang, Z. and Purves, D. (2004). The statistical structure of natural light patterns determines perceived light intensity. *Proceedings of the National Academy of Sciences of the United States of America*, 101(23):8745–8750.

Zhang, M. and Fulcher, J. (1996). Face recognition using artificial neural network group-based adaptive tolerance (gat) trees. *IEEE Transactions on Neural Networks*, 7(3):555–567.

Index

H

I

J

K

L

M

N

O

P

T

U

V

W

Z